Jenny Craig™

Diabetes Cookbook

Easy Homestyle Recipes for Healthy Living

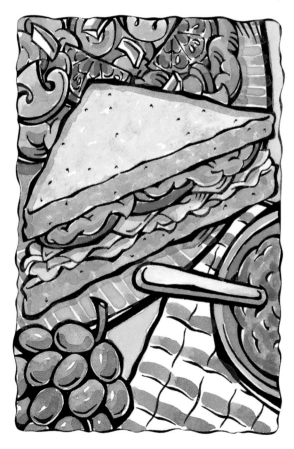

Oxmoor
House®

©1997 by Oxmoor House, Inc.
Book Division of Southern Progress Corporation
P.O. Box 2463, Birmingham, Alabama 35201

Library of Congress Catalog Card Number: 97-68655
ISBN: 0-8487-1803-8
Manufactured in the United States of America
First Printing 1997

Be sure to check with your health-care provider before making any changes to your diet.

Editor-in-Chief: Nancy Fitzpatrick Wyatt
Senior Foods Editor: Katherine M. Eakin
Senior Editor, Editorial Services: Olivia Kindig Wells
Art Director: James Boone

Jenny Craig™ Diabetes Cookbook
Easy Homestyle Recipes for Healthy Living

Editors: Anne Chappell Cain, M.S., M.P.H., R.D.;
    Cathy A. Wesler, R.D.
Jenny Craig, Inc. Contributing Editors: Jan Strode,
    Lisa Talamini Jones, R.D.
Copy Editors: Jaqueline Giovanelli, Shari K. Wimberly
Indexer: Mary Ann Laurens
Editorial Assistants: Stacey Geary, Andrea Noble
Illustrator: Susan Harrison
Senior Production Designer: Larry Hunter
Designer: Eleanor Cameron
Production Director: Phillip Lee
Associate Production Manager: Vanessa Cobbs Richardson
Production Assistant: Faye Porter Bonner

CONTENTS

Introduction

If you or someone you love has been recently diagnosed with diabetes, you are not alone. At least 16 million Americans share your condition, including 8 million who are undiagnosed. The good news is that there are many things you can do to succesfully manage diabetes. One of the most important is to begin eating healthier. This cookbook will show you just how easy it is to eat for both good health and great taste.

Today's approach to diabetes management is an individualized one. It's important to work with your dietitian or diabetes educator to create a plan that matches your personal tastes and lifestyle as well as your specific health concerns. These recipes will give you the flexibility to do just that. And, they can be enjoyed by everyone—friends, family, or anyone who enjoys delicious food.

All the recipes in this cookbook are low in fat and sugar. Most are sugar-free; some include small amounts of table sugar or other sweeteners. There are also plenty of low-cholesterol and low-sodium recipes. Regardless of your particular health needs, you'll have a variety of options from which to choose.

Do you need ideas for quick meals for everyday cooking? Or would you like a lightened version of an old family favorite? Whether you're a novice or a seasoned chef, you'll find many possibilities. Here's what to look for:

- Over 300 kitchen-tested homestyle recipes
- Familiar ingredients and easy cooking techniques
- Simple-to-make recipes that can be on the table in five steps or less
- Low-fat, reduced-sugar, and sugar-free recipes developed and tested by registered dietitians and culinary experts at the University of Alabama at Birmingham, *Cooking Light* magazine, and Oxmoor House
- Exchange lists from the *Exchange Lists for Meal Planning* developed by The American Dietetic Association and the American Diabetes Association
- Nutrient values for calories, carbohydrate, protein, fat, fiber, sodium, and cholesterol

For over 30 years, I have helped people recognize the lifestyle changes necessary for long-term weight management. In the process of losing weight, many have improved their health and have renewed their enthusiasm for living. It is my sincere hope that this cookbook will help you create your own healthy lifestyle, improve your control of diabetes, and enhance your health and well-being.

Jenny Craig

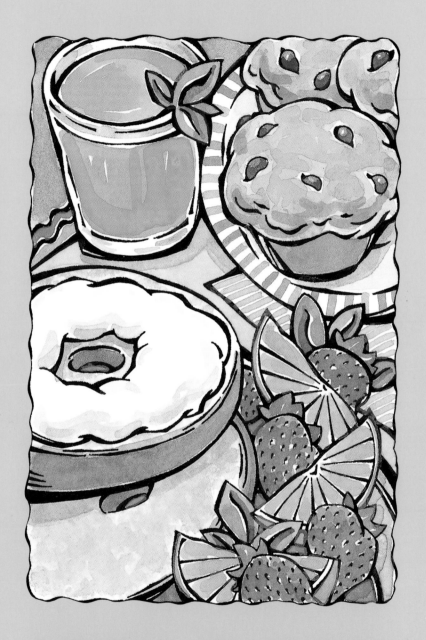

LIVING HEALTHY
WITH DIABETES

Living Healthy with Diabetes

Gone are the days of the "one size fits all" diabetes regimen. Experts now recommend an individualized plan, one that considers a person's lifestyle, eating habits, exercise patterns, and specific health concerns. The more you learn about your diabetes, the more flexibility you'll have in your daily choices. To stay healthy, it's best to keep blood glucose levels as near to normal as possible. Doing so may reduce the risk for complications like high blood pressure, nerve damage, and diseases of the heart, kidneys, and eyes.

What's Your Type?

Type I: Consistency

If you have Type I, or insulin dependent, diabetes (IDDM), aim for consistency in all things—meal schedule, number of meals, and the amount of carbohydrate eaten at each meal. This way, you may avoid the risk of either high or low blood sugar levels. Avoid skipping meals, which may sap both your energy and your blood glucose.

Type II: Weight Management

If you have Type II, or non-insulin dependent, diabetes (NIDDM), weight management may be the key to your health. At least 85 percent of people with NIDDM are overweight, and these same individuals have four times the usual risk for heart disease. Following a lower fat menu, moderating food portions, and becoming more physically active can help you maintain a reasonable weight and improve your blood glucose control. Weight loss through these simple lifestyle changes may even prevent or eliminate your need for medication.

Trade Diet for Lifestyle

Having diabetes doesn't mean following a rigid, restrictive diet. In fact, it doesn't mean dieting at all. Healthy eating, whether for weight loss or diabetes control, is not about deprivation. It's about balance, variety, and moderation. All foods can be part of a healthy meal plan—even one designed for a person with diabetes.

Why Weight?

Your weight can make a big difference in your health. If you have non-insulin dependent diabetes, losing weight can improve your blood glucose control and reduce your risk for a variety of diseases. Even a small weight loss—as little as 10 percent of your current weight—can result in significant gains in your control of diabetes, cholesterol levels, and blood pressure. And regardless of how much you lose, the switch to a lower fat menu with plenty of high-fiber grains, fruits, and vegetables, along with consistent physical activity, may reduce your risk for other serious health conditions such as heart disease and certain cancers.

Seven Strategies for Weight Success

1. Set reasonable weight goals—shoot for a loss of 1 to 2 pounds per week.
2. Focus on lowering your fat intake—balance your choices over several days.
3. Get physical—let a variety of fun activities help shape your daily routine.
4. Use the buddy system—a walking buddy or a low-fat cooking partner can be inspiring.
5. Build on the positive—learn from your lapses and reward your changes.
6. Never say never—commit to change, but aim for progress, not perfection.
7. Redefine success—energy, esteem, and health are benefits that can't be measured on the scale.

Body Mass Index

Body Mass Index (BMI) is a height-weight calculation that you can use to determine if your weight is in a healthy range. If you are overweight, BMI is a more accurate measurement of your body fat than the former "ideal" weights listed in life insurance weight tables. As a general guide, see the chart below. Your dietitian or diabetes educator can help you decide what is a reasonable weight for you.

To use the BMI table below, find your height in inches on the left side of the table. On the row corresponding to your height, find your current weight, then look at the numbers at the very top of the column to find your BMI. Use the table on page 9 to determine your health risk.

Body Mass Index

HEIGHT	19	21	23	25	27 WEIGHT	30	32	34	36	38	40
58"	91	100	110	119	129	143	152	162	172	181	191
59"	94	104	114	124	134	149	159	169	179	188	198
60"	97	107	117	127	138	153	163	173	183	194	204
61"	101	111	122	132	143	159	169	180	191	201	212
62"	103	114	125	136	147	163	174	185	196	206	217
63"	107	119	130	141	152	169	181	192	203	214	226
64"	111	123	135	146	158	176	187	199	211	223	234
65"	114	126	138	150	162	180	192	204	216	228	240
66"	118	131	143	156	168	187	199	212	224	236	249
67"	121	134	147	159	172	191	204	217	229	242	255
68"	125	139	152	165	178	198	211	224	238	251	264
69"	128	142	155	169	182	203	216	230	243	257	270
70"	133	147	161	175	189	210	224	237	251	265	279
71"	136	150	164	179	193	214	229	243	257	271	286
72"	140	155	170	185	199	221	236	251	266	281	295
73"	143	158	174	189	204	226	241	257	272	287	302
74"	148	164	179	195	210	234	249	265	281	296	312

Adapted from: Weighing The Options: Criteria For Evaluating Weight-Management Programs. Washington D.C.: National Academy of Sciences, 1995.

Body Mass Index and Health Risk

BMI	Risk
19–24	Healthy Weight
25–26	Low
27–29	Moderate
30–34	High
35–39	Very High
40+	Extremely High

Active Lifestyle

Physical activity is another important component of diabetes management and, in fact, offers you a host of health benefits. Exercise may reduce the risk for heart disease and certain cancers, lower blood pressure, improve blood cholesterol, help you maintain weight loss, and improve your blood glucose control. And all it takes is 30 minutes three to five days a week.

The trick is to accumulate exercise over the course of the day—take the stairs, work in the garden, walk at lunch, wash the car on the weekends. Every move adds up to better health. If you are on insulin or oral medication, consult with your diabetes educator on how to balance your physical activity with your medication and diet.

Log Your Successes

A lifestyle log or daily journal is an invaluable tool for diabetes control. A daily record helps you see how the foods you eat, your physical activity, and medication affect your blood glucose. It can also help you be more aware of stress and other factors that throw your blood glucose off balance. Not only will your log enable you to monitor your blood glucose trends, it can help you become aware of the many factors that drive your food and exercise choices. Use your log to track your progress, identify areas for change, and celebrate successes.

Nutrition Basics

The Jenny Craig Food Group Pyramid helps illustrate the appropriate balance of foods in your diet. It's similar to the United States Department of Agriculture (USDA) Food Guide Pyramid and communicates the same message: Eat less fat, and build your diet upon a base of complex carbohydrates. Both the Jenny Craig Food Group Pyramid and the updated *Exchange Lists for Meal Planning* are practical guides to balancing a variety of food choices in moderate amounts as part of your personal diabetes management plan.

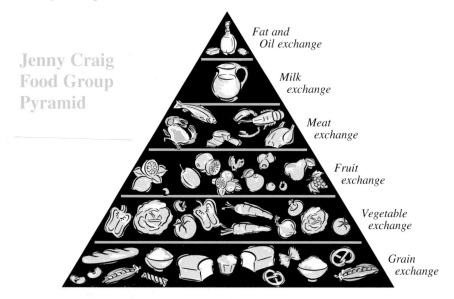

Jenny Craig Food Group Pyramid

Fat and Oil exchange

Milk exchange

Meat exchange

Fruit exchange

Vegetable exchange

Grain exchange

Cutting through the Fat

For optimum health, balancing your fat intake matters as much as keeping up with the number of calories or the amount of carbohydrate you eat. To find our how much fat you're consuming, check fat grams on the nutrition labels of the foods you purchase. Also, follow your blood fat levels. Depending on your blood fat profile, it may be helpful to modify the amount and kind of fat you eat.

To reduce your blood cholesterol, it's best to lower your fat intake to less than 30 percent of total daily calories, and avoid saturated fat from fatty meats, high-fat dairy products, shortening, and coconut and palm oils. Experts also advise reducing cholesterol intake to under 300 milligrams per day.

If your triglyceride level is elevated, you also may need to cut down on foods that are high in saturated fat (see list below). When making a selection from the Fat List, it's healthier to choose fats that are high in monounsaturates (see page 28). Losing weight can also help lower your blood triglyceride level. Your dietitian can advise you on the amounts and kinds of fat that are best for you.

Saturated Fat Sources

Saturated fat, found mainly in foods from animal sources and whole milk dairy products, can also be found in a few plant products.

Butter	Ice cream	Palm kernel oil
Cheese	Lard	Poultry (skin)
Coconut oil	Meats	Whole milk
Cream	Palm oil	

Carbohydrates: Relaxing the Rules

Nutrition guidelines regarding sugar intake for people with diabetes have been liberalized over the past few years. Research shows that it's the total amount of carbohydrate, rather than the type of carbohydrate, that is the critical factor affecting blood glucose control.

You can enjoy moderate amounts of sugar-containing foods, as long as you calculate them into your daily plan. (Be sure to discuss with your dietitian or diabetes educator the possibility of including sugar-containing foods in your nutrition plan.)

Carbohydrate Counting

Because of the greater emphasis on amount versus type of carbohydrate in meal planning, some people with diabetes count grams of carbohydrate to manage their blood glucose. With this system, instead of using the exchange lists, you count the carbohydrate grams in starchy foods like bread, dairy products, fruits, and vegetables, or sugar-containing foods like cookies and cake. You can work with your dietitian or diabetes educator to determine if this tool is for you.

Using the Exchange Lists

Exchange lists consist of foods separated into groups according to their nutritional similarities. Each serving of a food on an exchange list has about the same amount of carbohydrate, protein, fat, and calories. That is why any food on a list can be exchanged for any other food on the same list. For example, you can trade the slice of bread you might eat for breakfast for ½ cup cooked cereal. Each of these foods equals one starch choice.

How To Read Them

Foods are listed with their serving sizes, which are usually measured after cooking. When you begin, you should measure the size of each serving. This may help you learn to "eyeball" correct serving sizes.

The table on page 13 shows the amount of nutrients in one serving from each list. Most foods in the Carbohydrate Group have about the same amount of carbohydrate per serving. Vegetables are in this group but contain only about 5 grams of carbohydrate per serving.

Exchange lists provide you with many food choices (foods from the basic food groups, foods with added sugars, free foods, combination foods, and fast foods). This gives you variety in your meals. Several foods, such as dried beans and peas, bacon, and peanut butter, are on two lists. This gives you flexibility in putting your meals together. Whenever you choose new foods or vary your meal plan, monitor your blood glucose level to see how these different foods affect it.

The exchange lists beginning on page 14 are the basis of a meal planning system designed by a committee of the American Diabetes Association and The American Dietetic Association. Although designed primarily for people with diabetes and others who must follow specific diets, the exchange lists are based on principles of good nutrition that apply to everyone. (Copyright 1995 by the American Diabetes Association, Inc., and The American Dietetic Association.)

12

Exchange List Nutrient Values

Groups/Lists	Carbohydrate (grams)	Protein (grams)	Fat (grams)	Calories
Carbohydrate Group				
Starch	15	3	1 or less	80
Fruit	15	—	—	60
Milk				
Skim	12	8	0–3	90
Low-fat	12	8	5	120
Whole	12	8	8	150
Other carbohydrates	15	varies	varies	varies
Vegetables	5	2	—	25
Meat and Meat Substitutes Group				
Very lean	—	7	0–1	35
Lean	—	7	3	55
Medium-fat	—	7	5	75
High-fat	—	7	8	100
Fat Group	—	—	5	45

Other Carbohydrates

The exchange list "Other Carbohydrates" includes food like cookies, cakes, and ice cream. Each serving contains 15 grams of carbohydrate and is equivalent to a grain, fruit, or milk exchange. For our recipes, we've counted these foods in the starch or fruit group. During weight loss, you might do this as well to make sure you receive the protein, calcium, and other nutrients you need. Be sure to discuss how to include these foods in your nutrition plan with your dietitian.

Starch List

Cereals, grains, pasta, breads, crackers, snacks, starchy vegetables, and cooked beans, peas, and lentils are starches. In general, one starch is:
- ½ cup of cereal, grain, pasta, or starchy vegetable,
- 1 ounce of a bread product, such as 1 slice of bread,
- ¾ to 1 ounce of most snack foods (some snack foods may also have added fat).

One starch exchange equals
  15 grams carbohydrate,
  3 grams protein,
  0–1 grams fat, and
  80 calories.

Breads

Bagel	½ (1 oz)
Bread, reduced-calorie	2 slices (1½ oz)
Bread, white, whole wheat, pumpernickel, rye	1 slice (1 oz)
Bread sticks, crisp, 4 in. long x ½ in.	2 (⅔ oz)
English muffin	½
Hot dog or hamburger bun	½ (1 oz)
Pita, 6 in. across	½
Raisin bread, unfrosted	1 slice (1 oz)
Roll, plain, small	1 (1 oz)
Tortilla, corn, 6 in. across	1
Tortilla, flour, 7–8 in. across	1
Waffle, 4½ in. square, reduced-fat	1

Cereals and Grains

Bran cereals	½ cup
Bulgur	½ cup
Cereals	½ cup
Cereals, unsweetened, ready-to-eat	¾ cup
Cornmeal (dry)	3 Tbsp
Couscous	⅓ cup
Flour (dry)	3 Tbsp
Granola, low-fat	¼ cup
Grape-Nuts	¼ cup
Grits	½ cup
Kasha	½ cup
Millet	¼ cup
Muesli	¼ cup
Oats	½ cup
Pasta	½ cup
Puffed cereal	1½ cups
Rice milk	½ cup
Rice, white or brown	⅓ cup
Shredded Wheat	½ cup
Sugar-frosted cereal	½ cup
Wheat germ	3 Tbsp

Starchy Vegetables

Baked beans	⅓ cup
Corn	½ cup
Corn on cob, medium	1 (5 oz)
Mixed vegetables with corn, peas, or pasta	1 cup
Peas, green	½ cup
Plantain	½ cup
Potato, baked or boiled	1 small (3 oz)
Potato, mashed	½ cup
Squash, winter (acorn, butternut)	1 cup
Yam, sweet potato, plain	½ cup

Crackers and Snacks

Animal crackers	8
Graham crackers, 2½ in. square	3
Matzoh	¾ oz
Melba toast	4 slices
Oyster crackers	24
Popcorn (popped, no-fat-added or low-fat microwave)	3 cups
Pretzels	¾ oz
Rice cakes, 4 in. across	2
Saltine-type crackers	6
Snack chips, fat-free (tortilla, potato)	15–20 (¾ oz)
Whole wheat crackers, no-fat-added	2–5 (¾ oz)

Beans, Peas, And Lentils
(Count as 1 starch exchange, plus 1 very lean meat exchange.)

Beans and peas (garbanzo, pinto, kidney, white, split, black-eyed)	½ cup
Lentils	½ cup
Lima beans	⅔ cup
Miso*	3 Tbsp

Starchy Foods Prepared With Fat
(Count as 1 starch exchange, plus 1 fat exchange.)

Biscuit, 2½ in. across	1
Chow mein noodles	½ cup
Cornbread, 2 in. cube	1 (2 oz)
Crackers, round butter type	6
Croutons	1 cup
French-fried potatoes	16–25 (3 oz)
Granola	¼ cup
Muffin, small	1 (1½ oz)
Pancakes, 4 in. across	2
Popcorn, microwave	3 cups
Sandwich crackers, cheese or peanut butter filling	3
Stuffing, bread (prepared)	⅓ cup
Taco shells, 6 in. across	2
Waffle, 4½ in. square	1
Whole wheat crackers, fat added	4–6 (1 oz)

* 400 mg or more sodium per exchange

Fruit List

Fresh, frozen, canned, and dried fruits and fruit juices are on this list. In general, one fruit exchange is:

- 1 small to medium fresh fruit,
- ½ cup of canned or fresh fruit or fruit juice,
- ¼ cup of dried fruit.

One fruit exchange equals
15 grams carbohydrate and
60 calories.

(The weight includes skin, core, seeds, and rind.)

Apple, unpeeled, small	1 (4 oz)
Applesauce, unsweetened	½ cup
Apples, dried	4 rings
Apricots, fresh	4 whole (5½ oz)
Apricots, dried	8 halves
Apricots, canned	½ cup
Banana, small	1 (4 oz)
Blackberries	¾ cup
Blueberries	¾ cup
Cantaloupe, small	⅓ melon (11 oz) or 1 cup cubes
Cherries, sweet, fresh	12 (3 oz)
Cherries, sweet, canned	½ cup
Dates	3
Figs, fresh	1½ large or 2 medium (3½ oz)
Figs, dried	1½
Fruit cocktail	½ cup
Grapefruit, large	½ (11 oz)
Grapefruit sections, canned	¾ cup
Grapes, small	17 (3 oz)
Honeydew melon	1 slice (10 oz) or 1 cup cubes
Kiwi	1 (3½ oz)
Mandarin oranges, canned	¾ cup
Mango, small	½ fruit (5½ oz) or ½ cup

Nectarine, small	1 (5 oz)
Orange, small	1 (6½ oz)
Papaya	½ fruit (8 oz) or 1 cup cubes
Peach, medium, fresh	1 (6 oz)
Peaches, canned	½ cup
Pear, large, fresh	½ (4 oz)
Pears, canned	½ cup
Pineapple, fresh	¾ cup
Pineapple, canned	½ cup
Plums, small	2 (5 oz)
Plums, canned	½ cup
Prunes, dried	3
Raisins	2 Tbsp
Raspberries	1 cup
Strawberries	1¼ cups whole berries
Tangerines, small	2 (8 oz)
Watermelon	1 slice (13½ oz) or 1¼ cups cubes

Fruit Juices

Apple juice/cider	½ cup
Cranberry juice cocktail	⅓ cup
Cranberry juice cocktail, reduced-calorie	1 cup
Fruit juice blends, 100% juice	⅓ cup
Grape juice	⅓ cup
Grapefruit juice	½ cup
Orange juice	½ cup
Pineapple juice	½ cup
Prune juice	⅓ cup

Milk List

Most milk products are on this list. Cheeses are on the Meat List and cream and other dairy fats are on the Fat List. Based on the amount of fat they contain, milks are divided into skim/very low-fat milk, low-fat milk, and whole milk. This table shows nutrient amounts for one serving:

Milk Type	Carbohydrate (grams)	Protein (grams)	Fat (grams)	Calories
Skim/very low-fat	12	8	0–3	90
Low-fat	12	8	5	120
Whole	12	8	8	150

One milk exchange equals
  12 grams carbohydrate and
  8 grams protein.

Skim and Very Low-Fat Milk *(0–3 grams fat per serving)*

Skim milk	1 cup
½% milk	1 cup
1% milk	1 cup
Nonfat or low-fat buttermilk	1 cup
Evaporated skim milk	½ cup
Nonfat dry milk	⅓ cup dry
Plain nonfat yogurt	¾ cup
Nonfat or low-fat fruit-flavored yogurt sweetened with aspartame or with a nonnutritive sweetener	1 cup

Low-Fat *(5 grams fat per serving)*

2% milk	1 cup
Plain low-fat yogurt	¾ cup
Sweet acidophilus milk	1 cup

Whole Milk *(8 grams fat per serving)*

Whole milk	1 cup
Evaporated whole milk	½ cup
Goat's milk	1 cup
Kefir	1 cup

Other Carbohydrates List

You can substitute food choices from this list for a starch, fruit, or milk choice on your meal plan. Some choices will also count as one or more fat choices.

....

One exchange equals

15 grams carbohydrate, or
1 starch, or 1 fruit, or
1 milk.

....

Food	Serving Size	Exchanges Per Serving
Angel food cake, unfrosted	$\frac{1}{12}$ cake	2 carbohydrates
Brownie, small, unfrosted	2 in. square	1 carbohydrate, 1 fat
Cake, unfrosted	2 in. square	1 carbohydrate, 1 fat
Cake, frosted	2 in. square	2 carbohydrates, 1 fat
Cookie, fat-free	2 small	1 carbohydrate
Cookie or sandwich cookie with creme filling	2 small	1 carbohydrate, 1 fat
Cranberry sauce, jellied	$\frac{1}{4}$ cup	1½ carbohydrates
Cupcake, frosted	1 small	2 carbohydrates, 1 fat
Doughnut, glazed	3¾ in. across (2 oz)	2 carbohydrates, 2 fats
Doughnut, plain cake	1 medium (1½ oz)	1½ carbohydrates, 2 fats
Fruit juice bar, frozen, 100% juice	1 bar (3 oz)	1 carbohydrate
Fruit snacks, chewy (pureed fruit concentrate)	1 roll (¾ oz)	1 carbohydrate
Fruit spreads, 100% fruit	1 Tbsp	1 carbohydrate
Gelatin, regular	½ cup	1 carbohydrate
Gingersnaps	3	1 carbohydrate
Granola bar	1 bar	1 carbohydrate, 1 fat
Granola bar, fat-free	1 bar	2 carbohydrates
Honey	1 Tbsp	1 carbohydrate
Hummus	$\frac{1}{3}$ cup	1 carbohydrate, 1 fat
Ice cream	½ cup	1 carbohydrate, 2 fats
Ice cream, light	½ cup	1 carbohydrate, 1 fat
Ice cream, fat-free, no sugar added	½ cup	1 carbohydrate

Food	Serving Size	Exchanges Per Serving
Jam or jelly, regular	1 Tbsp	1 carbohydrate
Milk, chocolate, whole	1 cup	2 carbohydrates, 1 fat
Pie, fruit, 2 crusts	⅙ pie	3 carbohydrates, 2 fats
Pie, pumpkin or custard	⅛ pie	1 carbohydrate, 2 fats
Potato chips	12–18 (1 oz)	1 carbohydrate, 2 fats
Pudding, regular (made with low-fat milk)	½ cup	2 carbohydrates
Pudding, sugar-free (made with low-fat milk)	½ cup	1 carbohydrate
Salad dressing, fat-free*	¼ cup	1 carbohydrate
Sherbet, sorbet	½ cup	2 carbohydrates
Spaghetti or pasta sauce, canned*	½ cup	1 carbohydrate, 1 fat
Sugar	1 Tbsp	½ carbohydrate
Sweet roll or Danish	1 (2½ oz)	2½ carbohydrates, 2 fats
Syrup, light	2 Tbsp	1 carbohydrate
Syrup, regular	1 Tbsp	1 carbohydrate
Syrup, regular	¼ cup	4 carbohydrates
Tortilla chips	6–12 (1 oz)	1 carbohydrate, 2 fats
Vanilla wafers	5	1 carbohydrate, 1 fat
Yogurt, frozen, low-fat, fat-free	⅓ cup	1 carbohydrate, 0–1 fat
Yogurt, frozen, fat-free, no sugar added	½ cup	1 carbohydrate
Yogurt, low-fat with fruit	1 cup	3 carbohydrates, 0–1 fat

*400 mg or more sodium per exchange

Vegetable List

Vegetables that contain small amounts of carbohydrates and calories are on this list. Vegetables contain important nutrients, so try to eat at least two or three vegetable choices each day. In general, one vegetable exchange is:
- ½ cup of cooked vegetables or vegetable juice,
- 1 cup of raw vegetables.

If you eat one to two vegetable choices at a meal or for a snack, you do not have to count the calories or carbohydrates because they contain small amounts of these nutrients.

One vegetable exchange equals

5 grams carbohydrate,
2 grams protein,
0 grams fat, and
25 calories.

Artichoke
Artichoke hearts
Asparagus
Beans (green, wax, Italian)
Bean sprouts
Beets
Broccoli
Brussels sprouts
Cabbage
Carrots
Cauliflower
Celery
Cucumber
Eggplant
Green onions or scallions
Greens (collard, kale, mustard, turnip)
Kohlrabi
Leeks
Mixed vegetables (without corn, peas, or pasta)
Mushrooms
Okra
Onions

Pea pods
Peppers (all varieties)
Radishes
Salad greens (endive, escarole, lettuce, romaine, spinach)
Sauerkraut*
Spinach
Summer squash
Tomato
Tomatoes, canned
Tomato sauce*
Tomato/vegetable juice*
Turnips
Water chestnuts
Watercress
Zucchini

* 400 mg or more sodium per exchange

Meat and Meat Substitutes List

Meat and meat substitutes that contain both protein and fat are on this list. In general, one meat exchange is:
- 1 ounce meat, fish, poultry, or cheese,
- ½ cup beans, peas, or lentils.

Based on the amount of fat they contain, meats are divided into very lean, lean, medium-fat, and high-fat lists. This is done so you can see which ones contain the least amount of fat. The table shows the nutrients for 1 ounce of these foods:

Meat	Carbohydrate (grams)	Protein (grams)	Fat (grams)	Calories
Very lean	0	7	0–1	35
Lean	0	7	3	55
Medium-fat	0	7	5	75
High-fat	0	7	8	100

Very Lean Meat and Substitutes List

One exchange equals

0 grams carbohydrate,
7 grams protein,
0–1 grams fat, and
35 calories.

(One very lean meat exchange is equal to any one of the following items.)

Poultry: Chicken or turkey (white meat, no skin), Cornish hen (no skin)	1 oz
Fish: Fresh or frozen cod, flounder, haddock, halibut, trout; tuna, fresh or canned in water	1 oz
Shellfish: Clams, crab, lobster, scallops, shrimp, imitation shellfish	1 oz
Game: Duck or pheasant (no skin), venison, buffalo, ostrich	1 oz
Cheese with 1 gram or less fat per ounce:	
Nonfat or low-fat cottage cheese	¼ cup
Fat-free cheese	1 oz

Other: Processed sandwich meat with 1 gram or less
    fat per ounce, such as deli thin, shaved meats,
    chipped beef*, turkey ham   1 oz
    Egg whites   2
    Egg substitutes, plain   ¼ cup
    Hot dogs with 1 gram or less fat per ounce*   1 oz
    Kidney (high in cholesterol)   1 oz
    Sausage with 1 gram or less fat per ounce   1 oz

(Count as one very lean meat and one starch exchange.)
Beans, peas, lentils (cooked)   ½ cup
* 400 mg or more sodium per exchange

Lean Meat and Substitutes List

. . . .

One exchange equals
  0 grams carbohydrate,
  7 grams protein, 3 grams fat, and
  55 calories.

. . . .

(One lean meat exchange is equal to any one of the following items.)
Beef: USDA Select or Choice grades of lean beef
    trimmed of fat, such as round, sirloin, and flank
    steak; tenderloin; roast (rib, chuck, rump);
    steak (T-bone, porterhouse, cubed); ground round   1 oz
Pork: Lean pork, such as fresh ham; canned, cured,
    or boiled ham; Canadian bacon*; tenderloin, center
    loin chop   1 oz
Lamb: Roast, chop, leg   1 oz
Veal: Lean chop, roast   1 oz
Poultry: Chicken, turkey (dark meat, no skin),
    chicken (white meat, with skin), domestic
    duck or goose (well-drained of fat, no skin)   1 oz
Fish:
    Herring (uncreamed or smoked)   1 oz
    Oysters   6 medium
    Salmon (fresh or canned), catfish   1 oz
    Sardines (canned)   2 medium
    Tuna (canned in oil, drained)   1 oz
Game: Goose (no skin), rabbit   1 oz

Cheese:

4.5%-fat cottage cheese	¼ cup
Grated Parmesan	2 Tbsp
Cheeses with 3 grams or less fat per ounce	1 oz

Other:

Hot dogs with 3 grams or less fat per ounce*	1½ oz
Processed sandwich meat with 3 grams or less fat per ounce, such as turkey pastrami or kielbasa	1 oz
Liver, heart (high in cholesterol)	1 oz

Medium-Fat Meat and Substitutes List

One exchange equals

0 grams carbohydrate,
7 grams protein, 5 grams fat, and
75 calories.

(One medium-fat meat exchange is equal to any one of the following items.)

Beef: Most beef products fall into this category (ground beef, meatloaf, corned beef, short ribs, Prime grades of meat trimmed of fat, such as prime rib)	1 oz
Pork: Top loin, chop, Boston butt, cutlet	1 oz
Lamb: Rib roast, ground	1 oz
Veal: Cutlet (ground or cubed, unbreaded)	1 oz
Poultry: Chicken (dark meat, with skin), ground turkey or ground chicken, fried chicken (with skin)	1 oz
Fish: Any fried fish product	1 oz

Cheese: With 5 grams or less fat per ounce

Feta	1 oz
Mozzarella	1 oz
Ricotta	¼ cup (2 oz)

Other:

Egg (high in cholesterol, limit to 3 per week)	1
Sausage with 5 grams or less fat per ounce	1 oz
Soy milk	1 cup
Tempeh	¼ cup
Tofu	4 oz or ½ cup

High-Fat Meat and Substitutes List

One exchange equals
  0 grams carbohydrate,
  7 grams protein,
  8 grams fat, and
  100 calories.

(Remember these items are high in saturated fat, cholesterol, and calories and may raise blood cholesterol levels if eaten on a regular basis. One high-fat meat exchange is equal to any one of the following items.)

Pork: Spareribs, ground pork, pork sausage	1 oz
Cheese: All regular cheeses, such as American*,	
Cheddar, Monterey Jack, Swiss	1 oz
Other:	
Processed sandwich meats with 8 grams	
or less fat per ounce, such as bologna,	
pimento loaf, salami	1 oz
Sausage, such as bratwurst, Italian,	
knockwurst, Polish, smoked	1 oz
Hot dog (turkey or chicken)*	1 (10/lb)
Bacon	3 slices (20/lb)

(Count as one high-fat meat plus one fat exchange.)

Hot dog (beef, pork, or combination)*	1 (10/lb)

(Count as one high-fat meat plus two fat exchanges.)

Peanut butter (contains unsaturated fat)	2 Tbsp

*400 mg or more sodium per exchange

Fat List

Fats are divided into three groups, based on the main type of fat they contain: monounsaturated, polyunsaturated, and saturated. Small amounts of monounsaturated and polyunsaturated fats in the foods we eat are linked with good health benefits. Saturated fats are linked with heart disease and cancer. In general, one fat exchange is:
- 1 teaspoon of regular margarine or vegetable oil,
- 1 tablespoon of regular salad dressing.

Monounsaturated Fats List

One fat exchange equals
  5 grams fat and
  45 calories.

Avocado, medium	⅛ (1 oz)
Oil (canola, olive, peanut)	1 tsp
Olives: ripe (black)	8 large
green, stuffed*	10 large
Nuts	
almonds, cashews	6 nuts
mixed (50% peanuts)	6 nuts
peanuts	10 nuts
pecans	4 halves
Peanut butter, smooth or crunchy	2 tsp
Sesame seeds	1 Tbsp
Tahini paste	2 tsp

Polyunsaturated Fats List

One fat exchange equals
  5 grams fat and
  45 calories.

Margarine: stick, tub, or squeeze	1 tsp
lower-fat (30% to 50% vegetable oil)	1 Tbsp
Mayonnaise: regular	1 tsp
reduced-fat	1 Tbsp
Nuts, walnuts, English	4 halves

Oil (corn, safflower, soybean)	1 tsp
Salad dressing: regular*	1 Tbsp
reduced-fat	2 Tbsp
Miracle Whip Salad Dressing: regular	2 tsp
reduced-fat	1 Tbsp
Seeds: pumpkin, sunflower	1 Tbsp

* 400 mg or more sodium per exchange

Saturated Fats List†

One fat exchange equals
  5 grams fat and
  45 calories.

Bacon, cooked	1 slice (20/lb)
Bacon, grease	1 tsp
Butter: stick	1 tsp
whipped	2 tsp
reduced-fat	1 Tbsp
Chitterlings, boiled	2 Tbsp (½ oz)
Coconut, sweetened, shredded	2 Tbsp
Cream, half and half	2 Tbsp
Cream cheese: regular	1 Tbsp (½ oz)
reduced-fat	2 Tbsp (1 oz)
Fatback or salt pork††	
Shortening or lard	1 tsp
Sour cream: regular	2 Tbsp
reduced-fat	3 Tbsp

† Saturated fats can raise blood cholesterol levels.
†† Use a piece 1 in. x 1 in. x ¼ in. if you plan to eat the fatback cooked with vegetables. Use a piece 2 in. x 1 in. x ½ in. when eating only the vegetables with the fatback removed.

Free Foods List

A free food is any food or drink that contains less than 20 calories or less than 5 grams of carbohydrate per serving. Foods with serving sizes listed should be limited to three per day. Do not eat three servings at one time, however, because it could affect your blood glucose level. Foods listed without serving sizes can be eaten as often as you like.

Fat-Free or Reduced-Fat Foods

Cream cheese, fat-free	1 Tbsp
Creamers, nondairy, liquid	1 Tbsp
Creamers, nondairy, powdered	2 tsp
Mayonnaise, fat-free	1 Tbsp
Mayonnaise, reduced-fat	1 tsp
Margarine, fat-free	4 Tbsp
Margarine, reduced-fat	1 tsp
Miracle Whip, nonfat	1 Tbsp
Miracle Whip, reduced-fat	1 tsp
Nonstick cooking spray	
Salad dressing, fat-free	1 Tbsp
Salad dressing, fat-free, Italian	2 Tbsp
Salsa	¼ cup
Sour cream, fat-free, reduced-fat	1 Tbsp
Whipped topping, regular or light	2 Tbsp

Sugar-Free or Low-Sugar Foods

Candy, hard, sugar-free	1 candy
Gelatin dessert, sugar-free	
Gelatin, unflavored	
Gum, sugar-free	
Jam or jelly, low-sugar or light	2 tsp
Sugar substitutes**	
Syrup, sugar-free	2 Tbsp

** Sugar substitutes, alternatives, or replacements that are approved by the Food and Drug Administration (FDA) are safe to use. Common brand names include:

Equal (aspartame)	Sweet-10 (saccharin)
Sprinkle Sweet (saccharin)	Sugar Twin (saccharin)
Sweet One (acesulfame K)	Sweet 'N Low (saccharin)

Drinks

Bouillon, broth, consommé*
Bouillon or broth, low-sodium
Carbonated or mineral water
Club soda
Cocoa powder, unsweetened   1 Tbsp
Coffee
Diet soft drinks, sugar-free
Drink mixes, sugar-free
Tea
Tonic water, sugar-free

Condiments

Ketchup   1 Tbsp
Horseradish
Lemon juice
Lime juice
Mustard
Pickles, dill*   1½ large
Soy sauce, regular or light*
Taco sauce   1 Tbsp
Vinegar

Seasonings

(Be careful with seasonings that contain sodium or are salts, such as garlic or celery salt, and lemon pepper.)
Flavoring extracts
Garlic
Herbs, fresh or dried
Pimento
Spices
Tabasco or hot pepper sauce
Wine, used in cooking
Worcestershire sauce

*400 mg or more of sodium per choice

**FIRST BAPTIST CHURCH
GLADSTONE, OREGON**

Combination Foods List

Many of the foods we eat are mixed together in various combinations. These combination foods do not fit into any one exchange list. Often it is hard to tell what is in a casserole dish or prepared food item. This list of exchanges for some typical combination foods will help you fit these foods into your meal plan. Ask your dietitian for information about any other combination foods you would like to eat.

Food	Serving Size	Exchanges per Serving
Entrées		
Tuna noodle casserole	1 cup (8 oz)	2 carbohydrates, 2 medium-fat meats
Lasagna	1 cup (8 oz)	2 carbohydrates, 2 medium-fat meats
Spaghetti with meatballs	1 cup (8 oz)	2 carbohydrates, 2 medium-fat meats
Chili with beans	1 cup (8 oz)	2 carbohydrates, 2 medium-fat meats
Macaroni and cheese*	1 cup (8 oz)	2 carbohydrates, 2 medium-fat meats
Chow mein (without noodles or rice)	2 cups (16 oz)	1 carbohydrate, 2 lean meats
Pizza, cheese, thin crust*	¼ of 10 in. (5 oz)	2 carbohydrates, 2 medium-fat meats, 1 fat
Pizza, meat topping, thin crust*	¼ of 10 in. (5 oz)	2 carbohydrates, 2 medium-fat meats, 2 fats

Food	Serving Size	Exchanges per Serving
Pot pie*	1 (7 oz)	2 carbohydrates, 1 medium-fat meat, 4 fats
Frozen Entrées		
Salisbury steak with gravy, mashed potato*	1 (11 oz)	2 carbohydrates, 3 medium-fat meats, 3–4 fats
Turkey with gravy, mashed potato, dressing*	1 (11 oz)	2 carbohydrates, 2 medium-fat meats, 2 fats
Entrée with less than 300 calories*	1 (8 oz)	2 carbohydrates, 3 lean meats
Soups		
Bean*	1 cup	1 carbohydrate, 1 very lean meat
Cream (made with water)*	1 cup (8 oz)	1 carbohydrate, 1 fat
Split pea (made with water)*	½ cup (4 oz)	1 carbohydrate
Tomato (made with water)*	1 cup (8 oz)	1 carbohydrate
Vegetable beef, chicken noodle, or other broth-type*	1 cup (8 oz)	1 carbohydrate

*400 mg or more of sodium per serving

Fast Foods List †

Food	Serving Size	Exchanges per Serving
Burritos with beef*	2	4 carbohydrates, 2 medium-fat meats, 2 fats
Chicken nuggets*	6	1 carbohydrate, 2 medium-fat meats, 1 fat
Chicken breast and wing, breaded and fried*	1 each	1 carbohydrate, 4 medium-fat meats, 2 fats
Fish sandwich/tartar sauce*	1	3 carbohydrates, 1 medium-fat meat, 3 fats
French fries, thin*	20–25	2 carbohydrates, 2 fats
Hamburger, regular	1	2 carbohydrates, 2 medium-fat meats
Hamburger, large*	1	2 carbohydrates, 3 medium-fat meats, 1 fat
Hot dog with bun*	1	1 carbohydrate, 1 high-fat meat, 1 fat
Individual pan pizza*	1	5 carbohydrates, 3 medium-fat meats, 3 fats
Soft-serve cone	1 medium	2 carbohydrates, 1 fat
Submarine sandwich*	1 sub (6 in.)	3 carbohydrates, 1 vegetable, 2 medium-fat meats, 1 fat
Taco, hard shell*	1 (6 oz)	2 carbohydrates, 2 medium-fat meats, 2 fats
Taco, soft shell*	1 (3 oz)	1 carbohydrate, 1 medium-fat meat, 1 fat

†Ask at your fast-food restaurant for nutrition information about
  your favorite fast foods.
*400 mg or more of sodium per serving

Using Food Labels

Nutrition Facts on food labels can help you with food choices. These labels are required by law for most foods and are based on standard serving sizes. However, these serving sizes may not always be the same as the serving sizes in this cookbook.

◆ Check the serving size on the label. Is it nearly the same size as the serving size on your exchange lists? You may need to adjust the size of the serving to fit your meal plan.

◆ Look at the grams of carbohydrate in the serving size. (One Starch, Fruit, Milk, or Other Carbohydrate serving has about 15 grams of carbohydrate.) So, if one serving of cereal, for example, has 13 grams of carbohydrate, you can count that as one Starch serving in your meal plan.

◆ Note that Dietary Fiber and Sugars are listed under Total Carbohydrate. These values are included in the amount listed for Total Carbohydrate.

◆ Look at the grams of protein in the serving size. (One meat serving has 7 grams of protein.) If the food has more than 7 grams of protein, you can figure out the number of meat servings by dividing the grams of protein by seven.

◆ Look at the grams of fat in the serving size. (One fat serving has 5 grams of fat.) If one waffle has 15 grams of carbohydrate and 5 grams of fat, it counts as 1 Starch and 1 Fat.

◆ Ask your dietitian to help you use the information on food labels so that you can fit a variety of foods into your meal plan.

Nutrition Facts

Serving Size ½ cup (114g)
Servings Per Container 4

Amount Per Serving

Calories 90   Calories from Fat 30

	%Daily Value*
Total Fat 3g	5%
Saturated Fat 0g	0%
Cholesterol 0mg	0%
Sodium 300mg	13%
Total Carbohydrate 13g	4%
Dietary Fiber 3g	12%
Sugars 3g	
Protein 3g	

Vitamin A 80%	•	Vitamin C 60%
Calcium 4%	•	Iron 4%

* Percent Daily Values are based on a 2,000 calorie diet. Your daily values may be higher or lower depending on your calorie needs:

		Calories:	2,000	2,500
Total Fat	Less than		65g	80g
Sat Fat	Less than		20g	25g
Cholesterol	Less than		300mg	300mg
Sodium	Less than		2,400mg	2,400mg
Total Carbohydrate			300g	375g
Dietary Fiber			25g	30g

Calories per gram:
Fat 9 • Carbohydrate 4 • Protein 4

Using the Nutritional Analysis

A nutritional analysis for one serving of each recipe in this book appears below the recipe title and the exchange values. The nutritional analysis lists the portion size of one serving.

Nutrient values are listed in whole numbers. If a nutrient is analyzed to have a value of 0.5 or more, it is rounded up to a whole number. If it is found to be less than 0.5, then a trace amount of the nutrient is available. If a nutrient has no value in a recipe, 0 will be listed.

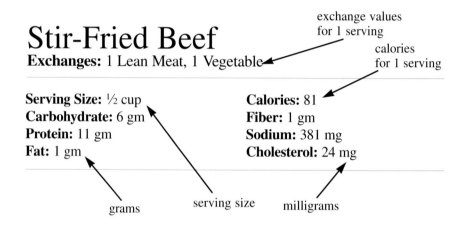

exchange values
for 1 serving

Stir-Fried Beef
Exchanges: 1 Lean Meat, 1 Vegetable

calories
for 1 serving

Serving Size: ½ cup
Carbohydrate: 6 gm
Protein: 11 gm
Fat: 1 gm

Calories: 81
Fiber: 1 gm
Sodium: 381 mg
Cholesterol: 24 mg

grams   serving size   milligrams

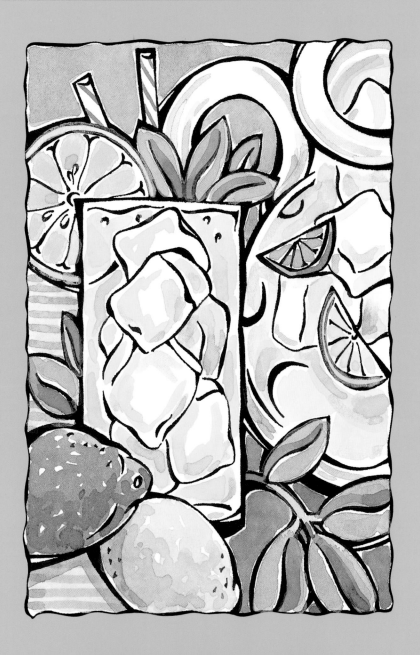

BEVERAGES

COCOA

Exchanges: 1 Skim Milk

Serving Size: 1 cup	**Calories:** 83
Carbohydrate: 13 gm	**Fiber:** 1 gm
Protein: 7 gm	**Sodium:** 252 mg
Fat: 1 gm	**Cholesterol:** 3 mg

INGREDIENTS:

2 tablespoons unsweetened
  cocoa
¼ teaspoon salt
1 cup water

3 cups skim milk
Sugar substitute to equal 8
  teaspoons sugar*
1 teaspoon vanilla extract

STEPS IN PREPARATION:

1. Combine cocoa and salt in a small saucepan. Add water, and place over low heat or in top of a double boiler. Boil gently, stirring constantly, 2 minutes.
2. Add milk and sugar substitute. Bring to a boil, stirring constantly; remove from heat immediately.
3. Stir in vanilla, and serve warm.

Yield: 4 servings

*See the sugar substitution chart on page 354.

SPICED HOT TEA

Exchanges: Free

Serving Size: ⅔ cup
Carbohydrate: 2 gm
Protein: trace
Fat: trace

Calories: 6
Fiber: 0 gm
Sodium: 5 mg
Cholesterol: 0 mg

INGREDIENTS:

4 cups water
1 cinnamon stick
3 whole cloves
Dash of ground nutmeg

2 thin lemon slices with rind
2 thin orange slices with rind
3 or 4 regular-size tea bags,
  as desired

STEPS IN PREPARATION:

1. Combine first 6 ingredients in a heavy saucepan; simmer 10 minutes.
2. Add tea bags, and let steep to taste. Remove tea bags, cinnamon stick, and cloves, and serve warm.

Yield: 6 servings

Use cinnamon sticks for hot beverage stirrers or float thin lemon slices on top for garnish and eye appeal.

LOW-CALORIE SPICED TEA MIX

Exchanges: Free

Serving Size: 1 teaspoon	**Calories:** 7
Carbohydrate: 1 gm	**Fiber:** trace
Protein: trace	**Sodium:** 1 mg
Fat: trace	**Cholesterol:** 0 mg

INGREDIENTS:

¾ cup sugar-free iced tea mix
¼ cup plus 2 tablespoons
  sugar-free orange-flavored
  drink mix
¼ cup sugar-free lemonade-
  flavored drink mix

2 tablespoons ground
  cinnamon
1 teaspoon ground cloves

STEPS IN PREPARATION:

1. Combine all ingredients, stirring until blended. Store mixture in an airtight container.
2. For each serving, place 1 teaspoon mix in a mug. Add 1 cup hot water, stirring well. Serve warm.

Yield: 72 servings

LEMON-ORANGE TEA

Exchanges: Free

Serving Size: ¾ cup
Carbohydrate: 6 gm
Protein: trace
Fat: trace

Calories: 25
Fiber: trace
Sodium: 10 mg
Cholesterol: 0 mg

INGREDIENTS:

½ cup boiling water
2 regular-size tea bags
Sugar substitute to equal 2
  tablespoons sugar*
1½ cups cold water
1 cup unsweetened orange
  juice

2 tablespoons lemon juice
1 (12-ounce) can sugar-free
  lemon-lime carbonated
  beverage

STEPS IN PREPARATION:

1. Pour boiling water over tea bags. Cover and let stand 5 minutes. Remove and discard tea bags. Transfer tea mixture to a medium pitcher, and stir in sugar substitute.
2. Add cold water, orange juice, and lemon juice. Cover and chill at least 1 hour.
3. Just before serving, add lemon-lime beverage to tea mixture, stirring well. Serve over ice.

Yield: 6 servings

*See the sugar substitution chart on page 354.

FRESH LEMONADE OR LIMEADE

Exchanges: Free (up to 4 cups per day)

Serving Size: 1 cup
Carbohydrate: 4 gm
Protein: trace
Fat: trace

Calories: 14
Fiber: 0 gm
Sodium: 8 mg
Cholesterol: 0 mg

INGREDIENTS:

¼ cup fresh lemon or lime juice
Sugar substitute to equal 4 teaspoons sugar*

1¾ cups cold water
Fresh mint leaves (optional)
Lemon or lime wedges (optional)

STEPS IN PREPARATION:

1. Combine juice and sugar substitute; add water, and stir well.
2. Serve over ice. If desired, garnish with mint leaves and lemon or lime wedges.

Yield: 2 servings

*See the sugar substitution chart on page 354.

APRICOT FIZZ

Exchanges: 1 Fruit

Serving Size: 1 cup
Carbohydrate: 18 gm
Protein: trace
Fat: trace

Calories: 72
Fiber: trace
Sodium: 15 mg
Cholesterol: 0 mg

INGREDIENTS:

3 cups unsweetened apricot
  juice, chilled
3 cups sugar-free ginger ale,
  chilled

1 tablespoon lemon juice

STEPS IN PREPARATION:

1. Combine all ingredients; stir well.
2. Pour into individual glasses, and serve immediately.

Yield: 6 servings

If unsweetened apricot juice is not available, you
can use unsweetened apricot nectar. Or try
unsweetened peach juice instead of apricot juice–
1 cup will still equal 1 Fruit Exchange.

CITRUS COOLER

Exchanges: 1 Fruit

Serving Size: 1 cup
Carbohydrate: 16 gm
Protein: trace
Fat: trace

Calories: 67
Fiber: trace
Sodium: 2 mg
Cholesterol: 0 mg

INGREDIENTS:

¾ cup boiling water
½ cup fresh mint leaves,
  coarsely chopped
4 cups sugar-free lemonade
1 cup unsweetened orange
  juice

1 cup unsweetened pineapple
  juice
¾ cup unsweetened grapefruit
  juice
Sugar substitute to equal ½
  cup sugar*

STEPS IN PREPARATION:

1. Pour boiling water over mint leaves. Cover and let stand 5 to 15 minutes. Strain mixture, discarding mint leaves. Transfer mint-flavored water to a large pitcher.
2. Add lemonade and remaining ingredients, stirring until blended. Cover and chill 2 hours.

Yield: 7 servings

*See the sugar substitution chart on page 354.

CRAN-ORANGE PUNCH

Exchanges: 1 Fruit

Serving Size: ½ cup
Carbohydrate: 11 gm
Protein: trace
Fat: trace

Calories: 47
Fiber: 0 gm
Sodium: 7 mg
Cholesterol: 0 mg

INGREDIENTS:

1¼ cups reduced-calorie
   cranberry juice cocktail
Sugar substitute to equal ¼
   cup sugar*
1 (6-ounce) can frozen orange
   juice concentrate, thawed
   and undiluted

2 cups sugar-free lemon-lime
   carbonated beverage

STEPS IN PREPARATION:

1. Combine cranberry juice, sugar substitute, and orange juice concentrate in a large bowl; stir well, and chill.
2. Just before serving, add lemon-lime beverage to fruit juice mixture. Serve over crushed ice.

Yield: 8 servings

*See the sugar substitution chart on page 354.

HOLIDAY PUNCH

Exchanges: ½ Fruit

Serving Size: 1 cup
Carbohydrate: 5 gm
Protein: trace
Fat: trace

Calories: 21
Fiber: 0 gm
Sodium: 17 mg
Cholesterol: 0 mg

INGREDIENTS:

3½ cups sugar-free lemon-
  lime carbonated beverage
2½ cups reduced-calorie
  cranberry juice cocktail

2 tablespoons lemon juice

STEPS IN PREPARATION:

1. Combine all ingredients in a punch bowl or pitcher.
2. Serve over ice.

Yield: 6 servings

Regular cranberry juice cocktail contains about
three times as much carbohydrate as reduced-
calorie cranberry juice, but both have essentially
the same amount of vitamin C.

TROPICAL FRUIT PUNCH

Exchanges: 1 Fruit

Serving Size: ½ cup
Carbohydrate: 12 gm
Protein: trace
Fat: trace

Calories: 47
Fiber: 0 gm
Sodium: 7 mg
Cholesterol: 0 mg

INGREDIENTS:

3 cups unsweetened
   pineapple juice
2 cups sugar-free lemon-lime
   carbonated beverage
½ cup unsweetened lime
   juice

Sugar substitute to equal ¼
   cup sugar*
2 teaspoons rum extract
Orange slices (optional)

STEPS IN PREPARATION:

1. Combine first 5 ingredients in a large pitcher; stir well.
2. Serve over ice, and garnish with orange slices, if desired.

Yield: 11 servings

*See the sugar substitution chart on page 354.

TROPICAL ICE

Exchanges: 1 Fruit

Serving Size: ½ cup
Carbohydrate: 13 gm
Protein: trace
Fat: trace

Calories: 53
Fiber: 1 gm
Sodium: 4 mg
Cholesterol: 0 mg

INGREDIENTS:

2½ cups unsweetened orange juice
2 cups mashed banana
Sugar substitute to equal 1 cup sugar*
1 tablespoon lemon juice

1 (20-ounce) can crushed pineapple in juice, undrained
1 (32-ounce) bottle sugar-free ginger ale
12 fresh strawberries (optional)

STEPS IN PREPARATION:

1. Combine first 5 ingredients in a large pitcher; stir well. Freeze until firm.
2. To serve, let stand at room temperature until partially thawed. Place in a punch bowl, and break into chunks. Add ginger ale, and stir until chunks soften. Garnish with fresh strawberries, if desired.

Yield: 24 servings

*See the sugar substitution chart on page 354.

PINEAPPLE-PEACH SMOOTHIE

Exchanges: 1 Fruit, 1 Skim Milk

Serving Size: 1 cup
Carbohydrate: 29 gm
Protein: 8 gm
Fat: trace

Calories: 144
Fiber: 1 gm
Sodium: 106 mg
Cholesterol: 3 mg

INGREDIENTS:

½ cup canned pineapple
  chunks in juice, undrained
½ cup unsweetened
  pineapple juice
2 canned peach halves in
  water, drained and diced

1 cup plain nonfat yogurt
1 cup skim milk
Sugar substitute to equal 2
  tablespoons sugar*

STEPS IN PREPARATION:

1. Combine first 3 ingredients in container of an electric blender or food processor; cover and process until pureed.
2. Add yogurt, milk, and sugar substitute; continue to process until smooth and thickened.
3. Pour into individual glasses, and serve immediately.

Yield: 3 servings

*See the sugar substitution chart on page 354.

CHOCOLATE-BANANA SHAKE

Exchanges: 1 Fruit, 1 Skim Milk

Serving Size: 1 cup	**Calories:** 129
Carbohydrate: 26 gm	**Fiber:** 1 gm
Protein: 7 gm	**Sodium:** 94 mg
Fat: trace	**Cholesterol:** 3 mg

INGREDIENTS:

2 cups skim milk
1 teaspoon unsweetened
   cocoa

1 medium banana, sliced

STEPS IN PREPARATION:

1. Combine all ingredients in container of an electric blender or food processor; cover and process until frothy.
2. Pour into individual glasses, and serve immediately.

Yield: 3 servings

ORANGE-YOGURT SHAKE

Exchanges: 1 Fruit, ½ Skim Milk

Serving Size: ½ cup	**Calories:** 91
Carbohydrate: 18 gm	**Fiber:** trace
Protein: 5 gm	**Sodium:** 54 mg
Fat: trace	**Cholesterol:** 2 mg

INGREDIENTS:

1 (6-ounce) can frozen orange juice concentrate, thawed and undiluted

1 cup skim milk
¾ cup plain nonfat yogurt

STEPS IN PREPARATION:

1. Combine all ingredients in container of an electric blender or food processor; cover and process until smooth.
2. Pour into individual glasses, and serve immediately.

Yield: 5 servings

Don't be confused by the amount of fat in yogurt. Low-fat yogurt contains 0.5 to 2 percent milkfat by weight; nonfat yogurt contains less than 0.5 percent milkfat. Both come in a variety of fruit flavors as well as plain.

STRAWBERRY-ORANGE SHAKE

Exchanges: 1 Skim Milk, ½ Fruit

Serving Size: 1 cup	**Calories:** 115
Carbohydrate: 18 gm	**Fiber:** trace
Protein: 9 gm	**Sodium:** 160 mg
Fat: 1 gm	**Cholesterol:** 5 mg

INGREDIENTS:

1½ cups skim milk
⅓ cup fresh strawberries
2 tablespoons unsweetened orange juice

Sugar substitute to equal 2 tablespoons sugar*
½ cup nonfat buttermilk

STEPS IN PREPARATION:

1. Combine first 4 ingredients in container of an electric blender or food processor. Cover and process until strawberries are pureed and mixture is frothy.
2. Transfer mixture to a small pitcher. Stir in buttermilk.
3. Pour into individual glasses, and serve immediately.

Yield: 2 servings

*See the sugar substitution chart on page 354.

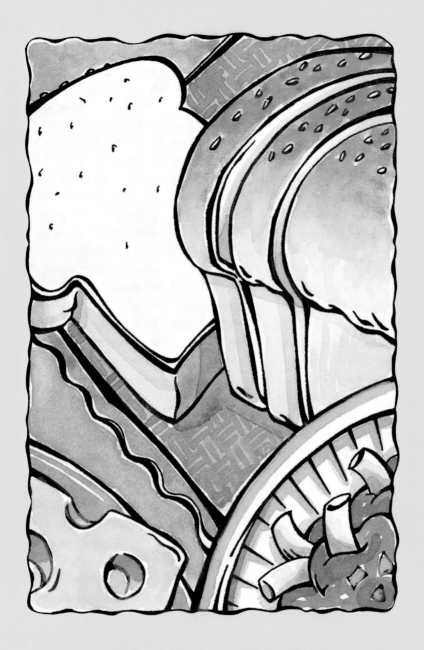

BREADS & CEREALS

FRESH CHIVE BUTTERMILK BISCUITS

Exchanges: 1 Starch

Serving Size: 1 biscuit	**Calories:** 60
Carbohydrate: 9 gm	**Fiber:** trace
Protein: 2 gm	**Sodium:** 110 mg
Fat: 2 gm	**Cholesterol:** 0 mg

INGREDIENTS:

2 cups all-purpose flour
1 tablespoon baking powder
¼ teaspoon baking soda
¼ teaspoon salt
½ teaspoon sugar
3 tablespoons chopped fresh
    chives

3 tablespoons margarine
¾ cup plus 1 tablespoon
    nonfat buttermilk
¼ teaspoon paprika

STEPS IN PREPARATION:

1. Combine first 6 ingredients in a medium bowl; cut in margarine with a pastry blender until mixture resembles coarse meal. Add buttermilk, stirring just until dry ingredients are moistened.
2. Turn dough out onto a lightly floured surface, and knead lightly 10 to 12 times. Roll dough to ½-inch thickness; cut into 21 rounds with a 2-inch biscuit cutter.
3. Place rounds on an ungreased baking sheet, and sprinkle with paprika. Bake at 425° for 10 to 12 minutes or until golden.

Yield: 21 biscuits

FRUITED SCONES

Exchanges: 1½ Starch, ½ Fruit, 1 Fat

Serving Size: 1 scone
Carbohydrate: 28 gm
Protein: 4 gm
Fat: 4 gm

Calories: 161
Fiber: 1 gm
Sodium: 153 mg
Cholesterol: 1 mg

INGREDIENTS:

2 cups all-purpose flour
1 tablespoon baking powder
¼ teaspoon baking soda
¼ teaspoon salt
1 tablespoon sugar
½ teaspoon grated orange rind

3 tablespoons margarine
½ cup diced dried mixed fruit
¾ cup nonfat buttermilk
1 tablespoon skim milk
Vegetable cooking spray
2 teaspoons sugar

STEPS IN PREPARATION:

1. Combine first 6 ingredients in a medium bowl, stirring to blend. Cut in margarine with a pastry blender until mixture resembles coarse meal.
2. Stir in dried fruit. Add buttermilk, stirring with a fork just until dry ingredients are moistened.
3. Turn dough out onto a lightly floured surface, and knead 10 to 12 times. Roll dough into an 8-inch circle, and cut into 10 wedges. Brush evenly with skim milk.
4. Transfer wedges to a baking sheet coated with cooking spray. Sprinkle evenly with 2 teaspoons sugar. Bake at 425° for 15 minutes or until golden. Serve warm.

Yield: 10 scones

APPLE MUFFINS

Exchanges: 1 Starch, ½ Fat

Serving Size: 1 muffin	**Calories:** 102
Carbohydrate: 17 gm	**Fiber:** 1 gm
Protein: 3 gm	**Sodium:** 226 mg
Fat: 3 gm	**Cholesterol:** 16 mg

INGREDIENTS:

1⅔ cups all-purpose flour
2½ teaspoons baking powder
½ teaspoon salt
Sugar substitute to equal 1
   tablespoon sugar*
1 teaspoon ground cinnamon
¼ teaspoon ground nutmeg

⅔ cup skim milk
¼ cup reduced-calorie
   margarine, melted
1 egg, lightly beaten
1 cup minced apple
Vegetable cooking spray

STEPS IN PREPARATION:

1. Combine first 6 ingredients in a medium bowl.
2. Combine milk, margarine, and egg; add egg mixture to dry ingredients, stirring just until dry ingredients are moistened. Fold in apple.
3. Spoon batter into nonstick muffin pans coated with cooking spray, filling two-thirds full. Bake at 400° for 25 minutes or until lightly browned.

Yield: 1 dozen muffins

*See the sugar substitution chart on page 354.

CARROT AND PINEAPPLE MUFFINS

Exchanges: 1 Starch, 1 Fat

Serving Size: 1 muffin	**Calories:** 127
Carbohydrate: 19 gm	**Fiber:** 1 gm
Protein: 2 gm	**Sodium:** 110 mg
Fat: 5 gm	**Cholesterol:** 15 mg

INGREDIENTS:

1¾ cups all-purpose flour
1 teaspoon baking soda
¼ teaspoon salt
1 teaspoon ground cinnamon
¼ teaspoon ground allspice
⅓ cup sugar
1 (8-ounce) can crushed pineapple in juice, undrained

1 cup shredded carrot
¼ cup vegetable oil
3 tablespoons skim milk
1 egg, lightly beaten
Vegetable cooking spray

STEPS IN PREPARATION:

1. Combine first 6 ingredients in a medium bowl.
2. Combine pineapple, carrot, oil, milk, and egg; add to dry ingredients, stirring just until dry ingredients are moistened.
3. Spoon batter into muffin pans coated with cooking spray, filling two-thirds full. Bake at 400° for 20 to 25 minutes or until lightly browned. Remove from pans immediately.

Yield: 14 muffins

RAISIN-BRAN MUFFINS

Exchanges: 1 Starch, ½ Fat

Serving Size: 1 muffin
Carbohydrate: 14 gm
Protein: 3 gm
Fat: 3 gm

Calories: 85
Fiber: 2 gm
Sodium: 214 mg
Cholesterol: 16 mg

INGREDIENTS:

½ cup all-purpose flour
1 teaspoon baking soda
2 cups wheat bran cereal
1 cup nonfat buttermilk
¼ cup reduced-calorie
　margarine, melted

Liquid sugar substitute to
　equal ¼ cup sugar*
1 egg, lightly beaten
¼ cup plus 2 tablespoons
　raisins
Vegetable cooking spray

STEPS IN PREPARATION:

1. Combine flour and soda in a medium bowl; add bran cereal.
2. Combine buttermilk, margarine, sugar substitute, and egg; add to dry ingredients, stirring just until moistened. Fold in raisins.
3. Spoon batter into muffin pans coated with cooking spray, filling two-thirds full. Bake at 400° for 18 to 20 minutes or until lightly browned.

Yield: 1 dozen muffins

*See the sugar substitution chart on page 354.

Wheat bran cereal is a good source of insoluble fiber. Health experts encourage Americans to aim for a total fiber intake of 20 to 35 grams per day.

CORNMEAL MUFFINS

Exchanges: 1 Starch, ½ Fat

Serving Size: 1 muffin
Carbohydrate: 16 gm
Protein: 3 gm
Fat: 2 gm

Calories: 91
Fiber: 1 gm
Sodium: 220 mg
Cholesterol: 16 mg

INGREDIENTS:

1 cup yellow cornmeal
¾ cup all-purpose flour
1½ teaspoons baking powder
½ teaspoon baking soda
½ teaspoon salt
Sugar substitute to equal 1
  tablespoon sugar*

1 cup nonfat buttermilk
2 tablespoons reduced-calorie
  margarine, melted
1 egg, lightly beaten
Vegetable cooking spray

STEPS IN PREPARATION:

1. Combine first 6 ingredients in a medium bowl. Mix lightly with a fork.
2. Combine buttermilk, margarine, and egg; stir well. Add to cornmeal mixture. Stir well; then beat gently for 1 to 2 minutes.
3. Spoon batter into muffin pans coated with cooking spray, filling two-thirds full. Bake at 400° for 25 to 30 minutes or until lightly browned.

Yield: 1 dozen muffins

*See the sugar substitution chart on page 354.

OATMEAL-BLUEBERRY MUFFINS

Exchanges: 1 Starch, 1 Fat

Serving Size: 1 muffin
Carbohydrate: 22 gm
Protein: 5 gm
Fat: 6 gm

Calories: 160
Fiber: 2 gm
Sodium: 201 mg
Cholesterol: 16 mg

INGREDIENTS:

2 cups regular oats, uncooked
1 cup plus 2 tablespoons all-purpose flour
1 tablespoon baking powder
½ teaspoon salt
Sugar substitute to equal 2 tablespoons sugar*

1 cup skim milk
¼ cup vegetable oil
1 egg
1 cup fresh blueberries
Vegetable cooking spray
1 teaspoon ground cinnamon

STEPS IN PREPARATION:

1. Combine first 5 ingredients in a medium bowl; make a well in center of mixture.
2. Combine milk, oil, and egg; add to dry ingredients, stirring just until dry ingredients are moistened. Fold in blueberries.
3. Spoon batter into muffin pans coated with cooking spray, filling two-thirds full.
4. Sprinkle cinnamon over muffins, and bake at 425° for 20 to 25 minutes or until lightly browned.

Yield: 1 dozen muffins

*See the sugar substitution chart on page 354.

TROPICAL MUFFINS

Exchanges: 1 Starch, 1 Fat

Serving Size: 1 muffin
Carbohydrate: 23 gm
Protein: 3 gm
Fat: 4 gm

Calories: 143
Fiber: 1 gm
Sodium: 237 mg
Cholesterol: 15 mg

INGREDIENTS:

1¾ cups all-purpose flour
2 teaspoons baking powder
¼ teaspoon baking soda
½ teaspoon salt
Sugar substitute to equal ¾ cup sugar*
¼ cup unsweetened shredded coconut
⅓ cup reduced-calorie margarine, melted

1 teaspoon grated orange rind
⅓ cup unsweetened orange juice
3 medium-size ripe bananas, mashed
1 egg, lightly beaten
Vegetable cooking spray

STEPS IN PREPARATION:

1. Combine first 5 ingredients in a large bowl; stir in coconut, and make a well in center of mixture.
2. Combine margarine, orange rind, orange juice, banana, and egg; add mixture to dry ingredients, stirring just until dry ingredients are moistened.
3. Spoon batter into muffin pans coated with cooking spray, filling two-thirds full. Bake at 375° for 25 to 30 minutes or until lightly browned.

Yield: 1 dozen muffins

*See the sugar substitution chart on page 354.

BANANA-APPLE BREAD

Exchanges: 1 Starch, 1 Fat

Serving Size: 1 (½-inch) slice
Carbohydrate: 21 gm
Protein: 3 gm
Fat: 4 gm

Calories: 123
Fiber: 1 gm
Sodium: 142 mg
Cholesterol: 23 mg

INGREDIENTS:

½ cup reduced-calorie
  margarine
Sugar substitute to equal 1 cup
  plus 2 tablespoons sugar*
2 eggs
1¾ cups all-purpose flour

2¾ teaspoons baking powder
1 cup peeled, coarsely
  chopped apple
3 medium bananas, chopped
Vegetable cooking spray

STEPS IN PREPARATION:

1. Cream margarine in a large bowl; gradually add sugar substitute, beating at medium speed of an electric mixer until light and fluffy. Add eggs, and beat until thick and lemon colored.
2. Combine flour and baking powder; add to creamed mixture, mixing well. Fold in apple and banana.
3. Spoon batter into an 8½- x 4½- x 3-inch loafpan coated with cooking spray. Bake at 350° for 65 to 70 minutes or until a wooden pick inserted in center comes out clean.
4. Cool in pan 10 minutes; remove from pan, and cool completely on a wire rack.

Yield: 1 loaf (16 slices)

*See the sugar substitution chart on page 354.

BLUEBERRY LOAF BREAD

Exchanges: 1 Starch, ½ Fruit

Serving Size: 1 (1-inch) slice	**Calories:** 108
Carbohydrate: 20 gm	**Fiber:** 1 gm
Protein: 3 gm	**Sodium:** 79 mg
Fat: 2 gm	**Cholesterol:** 0 mg

INGREDIENTS:

⅔ cup all-purpose flour
½ teaspoon baking powder
¼ teaspoon baking soda
Dash of salt
¼ cup sugar
¼ cup plus 2 tablespoons
   plain nonfat yogurt
2 teaspoons vegetable oil

½ teaspoon vanilla extract
1 egg white, lightly beaten
⅓ cup fresh or frozen
   blueberries, thawed
Vegetable cooking spray

STEPS IN PREPARATION:

1. Combine first 5 ingredients in a medium bowl.
2. Combine yogurt and next 3 ingredients; add to dry ingredients, stirring mixture just until dry ingredients are moistened. Fold in blueberries.
3. Spoon batter into a 6- x 3- x 2-inch loafpan coated with cooking spray. Bake at 350° for 35 to 40 minutes or until a wooden pick inserted in center comes out clean. Remove from pan immediately, and let cool on a wire rack.

Yield: 1 loaf (6 slices)

ZUCCHINI-ORANGE BREAD

Exchanges: 1 Starch

Serving Size: 1 (½-inch) slice
Carbohydrate: 17 gm
Protein: 2 gm
Fat: 2 gm

Calories: 93
Fiber: trace
Sodium: 45 mg
Cholesterol: 0 mg

INGREDIENTS:

1¾ cups all-purpose flour
2½ teaspoons baking powder
¼ teaspoon salt
½ cup sugar
1 teaspoon grated orange rind
1 cup finely shredded zucchini

½ cup unsweetened orange juice
⅓ cup frozen egg substitute, thawed
2 tablespoons vegetable oil
½ teaspoon orange extract
Vegetable cooking spray

STEPS IN PREPARATION:

1. Combine first 5 ingredients in a large bowl. Press zucchini between paper towels to remove excess moisture; add zucchini to dry ingredients.
2. Combine orange juice and next 3 ingredients, stirring well. Add orange juice mixture to zucchini mixture, stirring just until dry ingredients are moistened.
3. Spoon batter into an 8½- x 4½- x 3-inch loafpan coated with cooking spray. Bake at 375° for 40 to 45 minutes or until a wooden pick inserted in center comes out clean. Let cool in pan 10 minutes; remove from pan; let cool completely on a wire rack.

Yield: 1 loaf (16 slices)

CASSEROLE CHEESE BREAD

Exchanges: 1 Starch, ½ Fat

Serving Size: 1 wedge	**Calories:** 96
Carbohydrate: 15 gm	**Fiber:** 1 gm
Protein: 3 gm	**Sodium:** 223 mg
Fat: 3 gm	**Cholesterol:** 28 mg

INGREDIENTS:

1 cup all-purpose flour
1 cup whole wheat flour
1 tablespoon baking powder
½ teaspoon salt
Sugar substitute to equal 2
  tablespoons sugar*
1 tablespoon instant minced
  onion
½ teaspoon dried Italian
  seasoning

⅓ cup skim milk
¼ cup reduced-calorie
  margarine, melted
2 eggs, lightly beaten
Vegetable cooking spray
1 tablespoon grated
  Parmesan cheese

STEPS IN PREPARATION:

1. Combine first 7 ingredients in a medium bowl; make a well in center of mixture. Combine milk, margarine, and eggs; add to dry ingredients, stirring just until dry ingredients are moistened.
2. Spoon batter into a round 1½-quart casserole coated with cooking spray. Sprinkle with Parmesan cheese.
3. Bake at 400° for 25 to 30 minutes or until a wooden pick inserted in center comes out clean. Let stand 10 minutes before slicing.

Yield: 1 loaf (18 wedges)

*See the sugar substitution chart on page 354.

MEXICAN CORNBREAD

Exchanges: 1 Starch, 1 Fat

Serving Size: 1 wedge
Carbohydrate: 18 gm
Protein: 5 gm
Fat: 5 gm

Calories: 136
Fiber: 1 gm
Sodium: 327 mg
Cholesterol: 6 mg

INGREDIENTS:

1 cup self-rising cornmeal
1 cup (4 ounces) shredded
  low-fat process American
  cheese
1 cup whole kernel corn
1 cup skim milk
½ cup chopped onion
⅓ cup reduced-calorie
  margarine

2 tablespoons chopped
  jalapeño pepper
½ teaspoon garlic powder
1 (4-ounce) jar diced
  pimiento, drained
Vegetable cooking spray

STEPS IN PREPARATION:

1. Combine first 9 ingredients in a medium bowl, stirring well.
2. Pour batter into a 10½-inch cast-iron skillet coated with cooking spray. Bake at 350° for 45 minutes or until golden. Cut into 10 wedges, and serve warm.

Yield: 10 wedges

CRANBERRY-PECAN BREAD

Exchanges: 1 Starch, ½ Fat

Serving Size: 1 (½-inch) slice
Carbohydrate: 13 gm
Protein: 2 gm
Fat: 3 gm

Calories: 88
Fiber: 1 gm
Sodium: 206 mg
Cholesterol: 10 mg

INGREDIENTS:

2 cups all-purpose flour
1 teaspoon baking powder
1 teaspoon salt
½ teaspoon ground cinnamon
½ teaspoon ground nutmeg
1 egg
Liquid sugar substitute to equal 1 cup sugar*
½ cup water
⅓ cup unsweetened orange juice

¼ cup reduced-calorie margarine, melted
3 tablespoons white vinegar
1 teaspoon grated orange rind
1 cup coarsely chopped cranberries
24 small pecans, chopped
Vegetable cooking spray

STEPS IN PREPARATION:

1. Combine first 5 ingredients in a medium bowl.
2. Beat egg; stir in sugar substitute and next 5 ingredients. Add egg mixture to flour mixture, stirring just until dry ingredients are moistened. Fold in cranberries and pecans.
3. Spoon batter into a 9- x 5- x 3-inch loafpan coated with cooking spray. Bake at 350° for 1 hour or until a wooden pick inserted in center comes out clean.
4. Cool in pan 10 minutes. Remove from pan; cool overnight before slicing.

Yield: 1 loaf (18 slices)

*See the sugar substitution chart on page 354.

ORANGE MARMALADE NUT BREAD

Exchanges: 1 Starch

Serving Size: 1 (½-inch) slice
Carbohydrate: 14 gm
Protein: 2 gm
Fat: 2 gm

Calories: 84
Fiber: 1 gm
Sodium: 132 mg
Cholesterol: 11 mg

INGREDIENTS:

2 cups all-purpose flour
1½ teaspoons baking powder
½ teaspoon baking soda
¼ teaspoon salt
½ cup skim milk
Liquid sugar substitute to equal ½ cup sugar*
2 tablespoons reduced-calorie margarine, melted

1 teaspoon grated orange rind
1 egg, lightly beaten
½ cup low-sugar orange marmalade
¼ cup chopped pecans
Vegetable cooking spray

STEPS IN PREPARATION:

1. Combine first 4 ingredients in a medium bowl.
2. Combine milk and next 4 ingredients. Add milk mixture to flour mixture, stirring just until dry ingredients are moistened. Fold in marmalade and nuts.
3. Spoon batter into a 9- x 5- x 3-inch loafpan coated with cooking spray. Bake at 350° for 1 hour and 40 minutes or until a wooden pick inserted in center comes out clean.
4. Remove from pan, and let cool on a wire rack.

Yield: 1 loaf (18 slices)

*See the sugar substitution chart on page 354.

PARKER HOUSE ROLLS

Exchanges: 1 Starch

Serving Size: 1 roll	**Calories:** 75
Carbohydrate: 12 gm	**Fiber:** trace
Protein: 2 gm	**Sodium:** 114 mg
Fat: 2 gm	**Cholesterol:** 23 mg

INGREDIENTS:

3 cups all-purpose flour,
   divided
1 package dry yeast
Sugar substitute to equal 6
   tablespoons sugar*
¾ cup skim milk

⅓ cup reduced-calorie
   margarine
½ teaspoon salt
2 eggs
Vegetable cooking spray

STEPS IN PREPARATION:

1. Combine 1½ cups flour, yeast, and sugar substitute.
2. Combine skim milk, margarine, and salt in a saucepan; cook over medium heat until margarine melts. Cool to 120° to 130°. Add liquid mixture to flour mixture. Add eggs; beat at low speed of an electric mixer 30 seconds. Increase speed to high; beat 3 minutes. Stir in remaining 1½ cups flour to make a stiff dough.
3. Turn dough out onto a lightly floured surface. Knead until smooth and elastic (about 8 to 10 minutes). Shape into a ball; place in a bowl coated with cooking spray, turning to grease top. Cover and let rise in a warm place (85°), free from drafts, 1 hour or until doubled in bulk. Punch dough down; cover and let rest 10 minutes.
4. Roll dough to ¼-inch thickness; cut with a 2-inch biscuit cutter. Make a crease across each circle, and fold one half over. Gently press edges to seal. Place rolls on baking sheets coated with cooking spray. Cover and let rise in a warm place, free from drafts, until doubled in bulk. Bake at 375° for 15 to 20 minutes or until lightly browned.

Yield: 2 dozen rolls

*See the sugar substitution chart on page 354.

CINNAMON ROLLS

Exchanges: 1½ Starch, ½ Fat

Serving Size: 1 roll	**Calories:** 128
Carbohydrate: 25 gm	**Fiber:** 1 gm
Protein: 3 gm	**Sodium:** 131 mg
Fat: 2 gm	**Cholesterol:** 16 mg

INGREDIENTS:

4 cups all-purpose flour, divided
1 package dry yeast
Sugar substitute to equal ⅓ cup sugar*
1 cup skim milk
⅓ cup plus 3 tablespoons reduced-calorie margarine, divided

1 teaspoon salt
2 eggs
Vegetable cooking spray
Sugar substitute to equal ½ cup sugar*
2 teaspoons ground cinnamon
¾ cup raisins, divided

STEPS IN PREPARATION:

1. Combine 2 cups flour, yeast, and sugar substitute to equal ⅓ cup sugar.
2. Combine milk, ⅓ cup margarine, and salt in a saucepan; cook over medium heat until margarine melts. Cool to 120° to 130°. Add liquid mixture to flour mixture. Add eggs; beat at low speed of an electric mixer 30 seconds. Increase speed to high; beat 3 minutes. Add remaining 2 cups flour, stirring to make a stiff dough.
3. Turn dough out onto a lightly floured surface. Knead until smooth and elastic (about 8 to 10 minutes). Shape dough into a ball, and place in a bowl coated with cooking spray, turning to grease top. Cover and let rise in a warm place (85°), free from drafts, 1 hour or until doubled in bulk. Punch dough down; divide in half. Cover and let rest 10 minutes.
4. Roll each half of dough to a 12- x 8-inch rectangle. Melt remaining 3 tablespoons margarine; brush half of melted margarine over each rectangle.
5. Combine sugar substitute equal to ½ cup sugar and cinnamon; sprinkle half of cinnamon mixture over each rectangle. Sprinkle each with half of raisins.

6. Roll up rectangles, jellyroll fashion, beginning at long sides; press edges and ends together to seal. Cut each roll into 12 slices. Arrange slices in 9-inch round baking pans coated with cooking spray.
7. Cover and let rise in a warm place, free from drafts, 30 minutes or until doubled in bulk. Bake at 375° for 20 minutes or until lightly browned. Cool slightly; remove from pans, and serve warm.

Yield: 2 dozen rolls

*See the sugar substitution chart on page 354.

Spices aren't just for flavor. USDA (United States Department of Agriculture) scientists found that cinnamon, cloves, and tumeric helped improve blood sugar levels. The spices appeared to help insulin work more effectively in laboratory tests. Although more research is needed to understand just how much of these spices would be needed to help regulate blood sugar, the benefits are just another reason to enjoy their savory touch in your diet.

PEAR-PEPPER RING

Exchanges: 1 Starch

Serving Size: 1 slice
Carbohydrate: 18 gm
Protein: 3 gm
Fat: 1 gm

Calories: 93
Fiber: trace
Sodium: 114 mg
Cholesterol: 30 mg

INGREDIENTS:

1 medium-size ripe pear,
  peeled and diced
¼ cup water
1 package dry yeast
Sugar substitute to equal 2
  tablespoons sugar*
1 teaspoon salt

1 teaspoon freshly ground
  pepper
1 egg
3 cups all-purpose flour
Vegetable cooking spray
1 tablespoon skim milk
1 egg yolk

STEPS IN PREPARATION:

1. Combine pear and water in a saucepan; cover and bring to a boil. Reduce heat; simmer 10 minutes or until pear is tender. Drain.
2. Place pear in container of an electric blender; cover and process until smooth. Transfer pear to a bowl; let cool to 105° to 115°.
3. Sprinkle yeast over pear. Add sugar substitute and next 3 ingredients. Add flour, stirring to make a stiff dough.
4. Turn out onto a floured surface; knead until smooth and elastic. Shape into a ball; place in a bowl coated with cooking spray, turning to grease top. Cover and let rise in a warm place (85°), free from drafts, 1 hour or until doubled in bulk.
5. Punch dough down. Shape into a ball; place on a baking sheet coated with cooking spray. Press dough in center to make a hole 6 inches in diameter (dough should resemble a large doughnut). Cover and let rise in a warm place, free from drafts, 1 hour or until doubled in bulk. Cut ½-inch-deep slashes around top of loaf.
6. Combine milk and egg yolk; brush over loaf. Bake at 375° for 30 to 35 minutes or until loaf sounds hollow when tapped.

Yield: 1 loaf (18 slices)

*See the sugar substitution chart on page 354.

GARLIC MONKEY BREAD

Exchanges: 1 Starch

Serving Size: 1 slice	**Calories:** 80
Carbohydrate: 16 gm	**Fiber:** 1 gm
Protein: 2 gm	**Sodium:** 127 mg
Fat: 1 gm	**Cholesterol:** 0 mg

INGREDIENTS:

1 package dry yeast
1 cup warm water (105° to 115°)
3 cups all-purpose flour, divided
1 teaspoon salt
Vegetable cooking spray

1 tablespoon reduced-calorie margarine, melted
1 teaspoon dried parsley flakes
⅛ teaspoon pepper
1 clove garlic, minced

STEPS IN PREPARATION:

1. Dissolve yeast in warm water in a large bowl; let stand 5 minutes.
2. Combine 1½ cups flour and salt; add to yeast mixture, stirring well. Gradually stir in remaining 1½ cups flour to make a stiff dough.
3. Turn dough out onto a lightly floured surface; cover and let rest 10 minutes. Knead until smooth and elastic (about 8 to 10 minutes). Place dough in a bowl coated with cooking spray, turning to grease top. Cover and let rise in a warm place (85°), free from drafts, 1 hour or until doubled in bulk.
4. Combine margarine, parsley, pepper, and garlic, stirring well. Shape dough into 1½-inch balls, and dip each in margarine mixture. Layer balls of dough in a 10-inch ring mold. Cover and let rise in a warm place, free from drafts, 1 hour or until doubled in bulk. Bake at 375° for 25 to 30 minutes or until lightly browned.
5. Cool in pan 5 minutes; invert onto a serving platter, and serve warm.

Yield: 1 loaf (18 slices)

POTATO PANCAKES

Exchanges: 1 Starch, ½ Fat

Serving Size: 2 pancakes	**Calories:** 103
Carbohydrate: 16 gm	**Fiber:** 1 gm
Protein: 4 gm	**Sodium:** 378 mg
Fat: 3 gm	**Cholesterol:** 47 mg

INGREDIENTS:

3⅓ cups shredded cooked potatoes
2 eggs, lightly beaten
¾ cup skim milk
¼ cup chopped onion
2 tablespoons reduced-calorie margarine, melted

2 tablespoons all-purpose flour
1 teaspoon baking powder
1 teaspoon salt

STEPS IN PREPARATION:

1. Combine potato and eggs; stir well. Add milk and remaining ingredients; stir well. Let stand 10 minutes.
2. For each pancake, spoon ¼ cup batter onto a hot nonstick skillet. Brown on one side; turn and brown other side.

Yield: 16 pancakes

FRENCH TOAST

Exchanges: 2 Starch, 1 Medium-Fat Meat

Serving Size: 2 slices
Carbohydrate: 26 gm
Protein: 10 gm
Fat: 6 gm

Calories: 202
Fiber: 1 gm
Sodium: 578 mg
Cholesterol: 189 mg

INGREDIENTS:

2 eggs
2 teaspoons skim milk
¼ teaspoon salt

4 (1-ounce) slices white bread
Vegetable cooking spray

STEPS IN PREPARATION:

1. Beat eggs. Add milk and salt; beat until frothy.
2. Dip each bread slice into egg mixture, coating well.
3. Place bread slices in a large nonstick skillet coated with cooking spray. Cook 4 to 5 minutes on each side until browned.

Yield: 2 servings

If you want to increase fiber in your diet, switch from white bread and other highly processed wheat products to whole-grain breads and cereals.

FARINA AND FRUIT

Exchanges: 1 Starch

Serving Size: ¼ cup
Carbohydrate: 12 gm
Protein: 3 gm
Fat: trace

Calories: 62
Fiber: trace
Sodium: 119 mg
Cholesterol: 1 mg

INGREDIENTS:

1 cup skim milk
⅛ teaspoon salt
2 pitted dates, chopped
2 tablespoons farina, uncooked
¼ teaspoon vanilla extract

Sugar substitute to equal 2 tablespoons sugar*
1 teaspoon reduced-calorie margarine
⅛ teaspoon ground cinnamon

STEPS IN PREPARATION:

1. Combine first 3 ingredients in a saucepan; bring to a boil. Gradually stir in farina and vanilla. Reduce heat, and simmer, stirring constantly, 2 to 3 minutes or until thickened.
2. Remove from heat; add sugar substitute and margarine, stirring until margarine melts.
3. Spoon mixture into serving bowls, and sprinkle evenly with cinnamon. Serve warm.

Yield: 4 servings

*See the sugar substitution chart on page 354.

BAKED CHEESE GRITS

Exchanges: 1 Starch, 1 Medium-Fat Meat·

Serving Size: ¼ cup	**Calories:** 139
Carbohydrate: 15 gm	**Fiber:** 0 gm
Protein: 8 gm	**Sodium:** 675 mg
Fat: 5 gm	**Cholesterol:** 68 mg

INGREDIENTS:

1 cup quick-cooking grits, uncooked
⅓ cup skim milk
2 cups (8 ounces) shredded low-fat process American cheese
½ teaspoon hot sauce
½ teaspoon salt
3 eggs, lightly beaten
Vegetable cooking spray

STEPS IN PREPARATION:

1. Cook grits according to package directions, omitting salt.
2. Add milk and next 4 ingredients, stirring well after each addition.
3. Pour into a 1-quart casserole coated with cooking spray. Bake at 325° for 30 to 35 minutes until firm and lightly browned; serve immediately.

Yield: 10 servings

OATMEAL WITH RAISINS AND CINNAMON

Exchanges: 1 Starch

Serving Size: ½ cup	**Calories:** 68
Carbohydrate: 13 gm	**Fiber:** 2 gm
Protein: 2 gm	**Sodium:** 135 mg
Fat: 1 gm	**Cholesterol:** 0 mg

INGREDIENTS:

1½ cups water
2 tablespoons raisins
¼ teaspoon salt

⅔ cup quick-cooking oats, uncooked
1 teaspoon ground cinnamon

STEPS IN PREPARATION:

1. Combine first 3 ingredients in a saucepan; bring to a boil. Stir in oats and cinnamon.
2. Reduce heat, and simmer 1 minute or until water is absorbed.
3. Remove from heat, and serve warm.

Yield: 4 servings

Quick-cooking rolled oats are the same as regular rolled oats except that they are cut and rolled into smaller, thinner pieces. This helps cut the cooking time from 15 minutes for regular oats to 5 minutes for quick-cooking oats. Quick-cooking and regular oats can be used interchangeably in recipes. Instant oats in individual packages aren't interchangeable because they are precooked and dried and often contain sugar, salt, and flavorings.

APPLE-CINNAMON OATMEAL

Exchanges: 1 Starch, 1 Fruit

Serving Size: ½ cup
Carbohydrate: 25 gm
Protein: 3 gm
Fat: 1 gm

Calories: 120
Fiber: 3 gm
Sodium: 347 mg
Cholesterol: 0 mg

INGREDIENTS:

1½ cups water
¼ teaspoon salt
⅔ cup quick-cooking oats, uncooked
2 tablespoons raisins
1 teaspoon ground cinnamon

1 medium apple, peeled and grated
Sugar substitute to taste (optional)

STEPS IN PREPARATION:

1. Bring water and salt to a boil in a saucepan. Stir in oats and next 3 ingredients.
2. Reduce heat. Simmer 1 minute or until water is absorbed.
3. Remove from heat, and serve warm. Sprinkle with sugar substitute, if desired.

Yield: 3 servings

CORNBREAD DRESSING

Exchanges: 2 Starch, ½ Fat

Serving Size: ¾ cup
Carbohydrate: 29 gm
Protein: 6 gm
Fat: 3 gm

Calories: 174
Fiber: 2 gm
Sodium: 499 mg
Cholesterol: 17 mg

INGREDIENTS:

3 cups crumbled cornbread
2 cups fat-free chicken broth
1 cup soft breadcrumbs
1 cup finely chopped celery
¾ cup finely chopped onion

½ teaspoon salt
½ teaspoon pepper
½ teaspoon poultry seasoning
2 egg whites
Vegetable cooking spray

STEPS IN PREPARATION:

1. Combine first 9 ingredients in a medium bowl; stir well.
2. Spoon into an 11- x 7- x 2-inch baking dish coated with cooking spray. Bake at 350° for 45 minutes or until lightly browned and set.

Yield: 8 servings

To get soft breadcrumbs, rub fresh bread slices between your hands or crumble fresh bread in a food processor.

SPOONBREAD

Exchanges: 1 Starch, ½ Fat

Serving Size: ½ cup
Carbohydrate: 15 gm
Protein: 5 gm
Fat: 4 gm

Calories: 110
Fiber: 1 gm
Sodium: 364 mg
Cholesterol: 48 mg

INGREDIENTS:

1 cup cornmeal
1 teaspoon salt
1 cup water
2 cups warm skim milk

2 eggs, lightly beaten
3 tablespoons reduced-calorie margarine, melted
Vegetable cooking spray

STEPS IN PREPARATION:

1. Combine cornmeal and salt in a medium saucepan. Stir in water; gradually add milk, stirring until smooth.
2. Cook over low heat, stirring constantly, until thickened.
3. Spoon a small amount of hot cornmeal mixture into eggs; stir well. Add egg mixture to remaining hot mixture, stirring constantly. Add margarine; stir well.
4. Pour into a 1½-quart baking dish coated with cooking spray. Bake at 375° for 40 to 50 minutes or until lightly browned.

Yield: 8 servings

CHEESE STRAWS

Exchanges: ½ Starch, 1 Fat

Serving Size: 3 straws
Carbohydrate: 7 gm
Protein: 2 gm
Fat: 4 gm

Calories: 72
Fiber: 0 gm
Sodium: 184 mg
Cholesterol: 4 mg

INGREDIENTS:

1 cup all-purpose flour
½ teaspoon baking powder
½ cup reduced-calorie
   margarine
1 cup (4 ounces) shredded
   low-fat process American
   cheese

3 tablespoons cold water
⅛ teaspoon hot sauce

STEPS IN PREPARATION:

1. Combine flour and baking powder in a medium bowl; cut margarine and cheese into flour mixture with a pastry blender until mixture resembles coarse meal. Slowly add water and hot sauce to mixture. Stir with a fork until all ingredients are moistened.
2. Chill mixture 1 hour.
3. Divide dough into 48 equal strips or fill a cookie press and form 48 straws. Place on nonstick cookie sheets. Bake at 375° for 8 to 10 minutes or until lightly browned. Place on wire racks to cool.

Yield: 4 dozen cheese straws

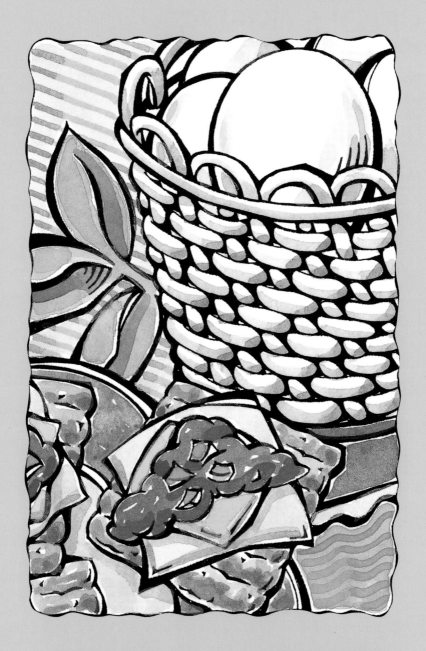

EGGS & CHEESE

CREOLE OMELET

Exchanges: 1 Starch, 1 High-Fat Meat, 1 Vegetable

Serving Size: ½ omelet	**Calories:** 191
Carbohydrate: 20 gm	**Fiber:** 3 gm
Protein: 10 gm	**Sodium:** 436 mg
Fat: 9 gm	**Cholesterol:** 221 mg

INGREDIENTS:

1 teaspoon vegetable oil
1 teaspoon all-purpose flour
½ cup thinly sliced onion
½ cup thinly sliced green pepper
½ cup thinly sliced celery
½ teaspoon dried thyme
1 clove garlic, minced
¼ cup canned no-salt-added chicken broth
1 (14½-ounce) can no-salt-added whole tomatoes, drained and chopped
¼ teaspoon salt
2 eggs, separated
1 tablespoon skim milk
1 tablespoon all-purpose flour
Dash of pepper
Vegetable cooking spray

STEPS IN PREPARATION:

1. Place oil in a medium nonstick skillet. Add 1 teaspoon flour; stir until smooth. Cook over medium heat until caramel colored, stirring often. Add onion and next 4 ingredients, and sauté over medium-high heat 4 minutes. Add broth, and cook until thick and bubbly, stirring often. Stir in tomato and salt. Set aside; keep warm.
2. Beat egg yolks in a small bowl at high speed of an electric mixer until thick and pale. Add milk, and beat until blended; set aside.
3. Beat egg whites at high speed of mixer until soft peaks form. Gradually add 1 tablespoon flour and dash of pepper, beating until stiff peaks form. Fold egg white mixture into yolk mixture.
4. Coat a nonstick skillet with cooking spray, and place over medium heat until hot. Pour egg mixture into skillet, spreading evenly. Reduce heat, and cook 8 minutes or until just set. Loosen omelet with a spatula; fold in half. Slide onto a serving platter. Spoon tomato mixture over omelet, cut in half, and serve immediately.

Yield: 2 servings

DEVILED EGGS

Exchanges: 1 Medium-Fat Meat

Serving Size: 2 egg halves
Carbohydrate: 1 gm
Protein: 6 gm
Fat: 5 gm

Calories: 70
Fiber: 0 gm
Sodium: 221 mg
Cholesterol: 187 mg

INGREDIENTS:

4 hard-cooked eggs, halved
2 teaspoons reduced-calorie
   mayonnaise
1 teaspoon vinegar
½ teaspoon dry mustard

¼ teaspoon salt
Dash of onion powder
Dash of pepper
Paprika

STEPS IN PREPARATION:

1. Remove egg yolks and mash. Set egg white halves aside.
2. Combine yolks, mayonnaise, and next 5 ingredients, stirring well.
3. Pipe yolk mixture into egg white halves. Sprinkle with paprika.
   Cover and chill.

Yield: 4 servings

The American Heart Association suggests that you
eat no more than four eggs each week to help keep
dietary cholesterol to a minimum.

EGGS BENEDICT

Exchanges: 1 Starch, 2 Medium-Fat Meat

Serving Size: 1 muffin half
Carbohydrate: 19 gm
Protein: 16 gm
Fat: 7 gm

Calories: 202
Fiber: 1 gm
Sodium: 657 mg
Cholesterol: 203 mg

INGREDIENTS:

2 whole English muffins
4 (1-ounce) slices lean cooked ham
1 medium tomato, cut into 4 slices
4 eggs, poached and kept warm

¼ cup plus 2 tablespoons plain low-fat yogurt
1 tablespoon lemon juice
1 teaspoon prepared mustard

STEPS IN PREPARATION:

1. Slice muffins in half, and toast.
2. Place 1 ham slice and 1 tomato slice on each muffin half. Broil 4 minutes.
3. Top each muffin half with 1 poached egg.
4. Combine yogurt, lemon juice, and mustard. Spoon 2 tablespoons yogurt mixture over each egg, and serve immediately.

Yield: 4 servings

BAKED EGGS AND MUSHROOMS

Exchanges: 1 Starch, 1 Medium-Fat Meat

Serving Size: ¼ recipe	**Calories:** 145
Carbohydrate: 17 gm	**Fiber:** 1 gm
Protein: 8 gm	**Sodium:** 375 mg
Fat: 5 gm	**Cholesterol:** 188 mg

INGREDIENTS:

4 eggs, lightly beaten
½ cup skim milk
⅛ teaspoon salt
Dash of pepper
1 cup cooked long-grain rice
  (cooked without salt or fat)

¼ cup canned sliced
  mushrooms, drained
Vegetable cooking spray
Cheese Sauce (page 290)

STEPS IN PREPARATION:

1. Combine first 4 ingredients; stir well. Stir in rice and mushrooms.
2. Pour into an 8-inch square baking dish coated with cooking spray. Bake at 350° for 30 to 35 minutes or until lightly browned and set.
3. To serve, cut into 4 equal portions, and serve with Cheese Sauce.

Yield: 4 servings

Store eggs in the shells for up to five weeks in the refrigerator. Keep them in the carton with large ends up to keep the yolks centered.

CHEDDAR-POTATO FRITTATA

Exchanges: ½ Starch, 1 Lean Meat

Serving Size: 1 wedge
Carbohydrate: 11 gm
Protein: 10 gm
Fat: 2 gm

Calories: 100
Fiber: 1 gm
Sodium: 263 mg
Cholesterol: 6 mg

INGREDIENTS:

1½ cups coarsely chopped
   round red potato
Vegetable cooking spray
1 cup chopped tomato
¼ cup chopped green onions
½ teaspoon pepper
¼ teaspoon salt
1½ cups frozen egg substitute,
   thawed

½ cup (2 ounces) shredded
   reduced-fat sharp Cheddar
   cheese

STEPS IN PREPARATION:

1. Cook potato in a saucepan in boiling water to cover 10 to 12 minutes or until tender. Drain well.
2. Coat a large nonstick skillet with cooking spray; place over medium-high heat until hot. Add potato, tomato, and next 3 ingredients; sauté until onion is tender.
3. Pour egg substitute over vegetable mixture. Cover; cook over medium-low heat 15 minutes or until set. Sprinkle with cheese. Cover; cook 2 minutes or until cheese melts. Cut into 6 wedges, and serve immediately.

Yield: 6 servings

Egg substitutes can be used in place of whole eggs in many recipes. One-fourth cup egg substitute is equivalent to one whole egg.

DEVILED EGG CASSEROLE

Exchanges: ½ Starch, 1½ Medium-Fat Meat

Serving Size: 2 egg halves
Carbohydrate: 9 gm
Protein: 11 gm
Fat: 8 gm

Calories: 152
Fiber: 0 gm
Sodium: 581 mg
Cholesterol: 195 mg

INGREDIENTS:

8 hard-cooked eggs, halved
½ cup reduced-calorie mayonnaise
¼ cup chopped mushrooms
¼ teaspoon salt
Vegetable cooking spray
2 tablespoons reduced-calorie margarine
2 tablespoons all-purpose flour

1½ cups skim milk
½ teaspoon Worcestershire sauce
1 cup (4 ounces) shredded low-fat process American cheese
Paprika

STEPS IN PREPARATION:

1. Remove egg yolks, and mash. Set egg white halves aside.
2. Combine yolks, mayonnaise, mushrooms, and salt.
3. Pipe yolk mixture into egg white halves. Place halves, cut side up, in a 2-quart casserole coated with cooking spray.
4. Melt margarine in a nonstick skillet; add flour, stirring until smooth. Gradually add milk and Worcestershire sauce, stirring constantly. Add cheese, stirring until cheese melts.
5. Pour cheese mixture over eggs; sprinkle with paprika. Bake at 350° for 30 minutes or until bubbly.

Yield: 8 servings

WESTERN-EGG CASSEROLE

Exchanges: 1 Starch, 1 Medium-Fat Meat

Serving Size: ¾ cup	**Calories:** 154
Carbohydrate: 18 gm	**Fiber:** 2 gm
Protein: 8 gm	**Sodium:** 457 mg
Fat: 5 gm	**Cholesterol:** 144 mg

INGREDIENTS:

1½ cups sliced celery
1 cup chopped green pepper
1 medium onion, sliced
1 tablespoon reduced-calorie margarine, melted
1 tablespoon all-purpose flour
1 teaspoon salt
1 (16-ounce) can low-sodium whole tomatoes, undrained

¼ teaspoon hot sauce
6 hard-cooked eggs, chopped
2 cups cooked long-grain rice (cooked without salt or fat)
Vegetable cooking spray
½ cup (2 ounces) shredded low-fat process American cheese

STEPS IN PREPARATION:

1. Sauté celery, green pepper, and onion in margarine in a 3-quart saucepan until vegetables are tender. Add flour and salt, stirring to blend.
2. Stir in tomatoes and hot sauce; bring to a boil. Reduce heat, and simmer, uncovered, 10 minutes or until mixture is thickened and bubbly, stirring occasionally. Carefully stir in chopped eggs.
3. Spoon rice into a 2-quart casserole coated with cooking spray. Pour egg mixture over rice, and bake, uncovered, at 350° for 25 to 30 minutes or until thoroughly heated. Top with cheese, and bake an additional 5 minutes.

Yield: 8 servings

EGG-RICE CASSEROLE

Exchanges: 1 Starch, 1 Medium-Fat Meat

Serving Size: ⅛ recipe
Carbohydrate: 17 gm
Protein: 7 gm
Fat: 4 gm

Calories: 135
Fiber: 1 gm
Sodium: 410 mg
Cholesterol: 164 mg

INGREDIENTS:

7 eggs, lightly beaten
¾ cup skim milk
½ teaspoon celery salt
Dash of pepper
2 cups cooked long-grain rice
  (cooked without salt or fat)

1 (4½-ounce) jar sliced
  mushrooms, drained
Vegetable cooking spray

STEPS IN PREPARATION:

1. Combine first 4 ingredients in a large bowl; stir well. Stir in rice and mushrooms.
2. Pour into an 11- x 7- x 2-inch baking dish coated with cooking spray. Bake at 350° for 30 to 35 minutes or until set. To serve, cut into 8 equal portions.

Yield: 8 servings

Don't wash eggs before storing because washing removes the protective coating that keeps bacteria out of the egg.

HAM OMELET

Exchanges: 2 Medium-Fat Meat

Serving Size: ⅕ omelet
Carbohydrate: 4 gm
Protein: 12 gm
Fat: 9 gm

Calories: 145
Fiber: 1 gm
Sodium: 462 mg
Cholesterol: 305 mg

INGREDIENTS:

8 eggs
½ cup skim milk
1 teaspoon Italian seasoning
½ teaspoon salt
½ teaspoon pepper
½ teaspoon hot sauce

1 tablespoon reduced-calorie
    margarine
1 medium tomato, chopped
⅓ cup finely chopped lean
    cooked ham

STEPS IN PREPARATION:

1. Beat first 6 ingredients with a fork until blended (do not overbeat).
2. Melt margarine in a medium nonstick skillet or omelet pan; add egg mixture. As mixture starts to cook, gently lift edges of omelet with a spatula, and tilt pan so uncooked portion flows underneath.
3. When egg mixture is almost set, spoon tomato and ham over half of omelet; continue cooking until eggs are set.
4. Loosen omelet with a spatula, and fold in half; slide onto a serving platter. Divide into 5 equal portions, and serve immediately.

Yield: 5 servings

POTATO-MUSHROOM OMELET

Exchanges: 1 Starch, 1½ Medium-Fat Meat

Serving Size: ¼ omelet
Carbohydrate: 14 gm
Protein: 14 gm
Fat: 7 gm

Calories: 174
Fiber: 1 gm
Sodium: 598 mg
Cholesterol: 195 mg

INGREDIENTS:

1 large baking potato, peeled and diced
Vegetable cooking spray
½ cup sliced fresh mushrooms
½ cup sliced green onions
4 eggs
4 egg whites
½ cup skim milk
½ teaspoon salt
¼ teaspoon pepper
½ cup (2 ounces) shredded low-fat process American cheese

STEPS IN PREPARATION:

1. Place diced potato in a small saucepan; add boiling water to cover. Cover and cook 10 minutes. Drain well.
2. Coat a 10-inch skillet with cooking spray; place over medium heat until hot. Sauté potato 5 minutes. Add mushrooms and onions, and sauté an additional 5 minutes or until vegetables are tender. Spread potato mixture in bottom of a 9-inch square baking dish coated with cooking spray.
3. Combine eggs and egg whites in a large bowl; beat at medium speed of an electric mixer until frothy. Add milk, salt, and pepper, beating until very light and fluffy.
4. Pour egg mixture over potato mixture, and bake at 350° for 20 to 25 minutes or until lightly browned and puffy. Remove from oven, and top with cheese. Serve immediately.

Yield: 4 servings

COTTAGE CHEESE OMELET

Exchanges: 1 Lean Meat

Serving Size: ½ omelet	**Calories:** 61
Carbohydrate: 1 gm	**Fiber:** trace
Protein: 8 gm	**Sodium:** 667 mg
Fat: 2 gm	**Cholesterol:** 95 mg

INGREDIENTS:

1 egg
2 egg whites
1 tablespoon water
1 teaspoon dried parsley
  flakes
½ teaspoon salt

¼ teaspoon dried marjoram
¼ teaspoon pepper
Vegetable cooking spray
2 tablespoons 1% low-fat
  cottage cheese

STEPS IN PREPARATION:

1. Combine first 7 ingredients in a small bowl, stirring well.
2. Coat a small nonstick skillet with cooking spray; place over medium heat until hot. Pour egg mixture into pan. As mixture starts to cook, gently lift edges of omelet with a spatula, and tilt pan so uncooked portion flows underneath.
3. When egg mixture is almost set, spoon cottage cheese over half of omelet; continue cooking until eggs are set.
4. Loosen omelet with a spatula, and fold in half; slide onto a serving platter, and serve immediately.

Yield: 2 servings

You can refrigerate leftover egg whites and egg yolks. Use raw egg whites within four days and raw egg yolks within one to two days.

CHEESE SOUFFLÉ

Exchanges: 1 Starch, 1 Medium-Fat Meat

Serving Size: ⅓ cup
Carbohydrate: 12 gm
Protein: 10 gm
Fat: 8 gm

Calories: 154
Fiber: 0 gm
Sodium: 631 mg
Cholesterol: 105 mg

INGREDIENTS:

4 (1-ounce) slices white
  bread, cubed
¾ cup skim milk
1 cup (4 ounces) shredded
  low-fat process American
  cheese
2 tablespoons reduced-calorie
  margarine

½ teaspoon salt
½ teaspoon Worcestershire
  sauce
Dash of ground red pepper
3 eggs, separated
Vegetable cooking spray

STEPS IN PREPARATION:

1. Combine bread and milk in a heavy saucepan; bring mixture to a boil. Add cheese and next 4 ingredients.
2. Beat egg yolks; gradually stir about one-fourth of cheese mixture into egg yolks. Stir egg yolk mixture into remaining cheese mixture.
3. Beat egg whites, and fold into cheese mixture.
4. Place mixture in a 1-quart casserole coated with cooking spray; place casserole in a pan of water. Bake at 400° for 35 to 40 minutes or until lightly browned; serve immediately.

Yield: 6 servings

EGGPLANT SOUFFLÉ

Exchanges: 1 Vegetable, 1 Medium-Fat Meat

Serving Size: ½ cup
Carbohydrate: 5 gm
Protein: 7 gm
Fat: 5 gm

Calories: 88
Fiber: 1 gm
Sodium: 395 mg
Cholesterol: 78 mg

INGREDIENTS:

3 cups diced eggplant
½ teaspoon salt
1 cup (4 ounces) shredded
low-fat process American
cheese
1 cup skim milk

1 tablespoon reduced-calorie
margarine
⅛ teaspoon hot sauce
Dash of pepper
3 eggs, lightly beaten
Vegetable cooking spray

STEPS IN PREPARATION:

1. Place eggplant in a saucepan with water to cover. Add salt, and cook 8 to 10 minutes or until tender. Drain and cool.
2. Add cheese and next 5 ingredients.
3. Place mixture in a 2-quart casserole coated with cooking spray. Bake at 350° for 30 minutes; serve immediately.

Yield: 8 servings

If you like eggplant, venture beyond the familiar dark purple variety. Several other varieties are also available. Italian eggplant is shaped the same as the standard type but has a delicate skin and fine flesh. White eggplant is usually less bitter than purple eggplant. Slender and straight, Oriental eggplant is often sweeter and smaller than the standard variety.

SPINACH SOUFFLÉ

Exchanges: ½ Medium-Fat Meat, 1 Vegetable

Serving Size: ½ cup	**Calories:** 79
Carbohydrate: 5 gm	**Fiber:** trace
Protein: 6 gm	**Sodium:** 298 mg
Fat: 4 gm	**Cholesterol:** 51 mg

INGREDIENTS:

Vegetable cooking spray
1 tablespoon grated
  Parmesan cheese
2 tablespoons reduced-calorie
  margarine
2 tablespoons all-purpose
  flour
1 cup skim milk
1 teaspoon instant minced
  onion
¼ teaspoon salt

¼ teaspoon hot sauce
⅛ teaspoon ground nutmeg
2 eggs, separated
1 (10-ounce) package frozen
  chopped spinach, thawed
  and well drained
½ cup (2 ounces) shredded
  low-fat process American
  cheese
2 egg whites
¾ teaspoon cream of tartar

STEPS IN PREPARATION:

1. Coat bottom of a 2-quart soufflé dish with cooking spray; dust with Parmesan cheese, and set aside.
2. Melt margarine in a 3-quart saucepan over low heat; add flour, stirring until smooth. Cook, stirring constantly, 2 minutes.
3. Gradually add milk and next 4 ingredients; cook over medium heat, stirring constantly, until thickened and bubbly. Remove from heat.
4. Place egg yolks in a small bowl; beat at medium speed of an electric mixer until thick and lemon colored. Gradually stir one-fourth of hot white sauce into egg yolks; stir egg yolk mixture into remaining white sauce. Stir in spinach and shredded cheese. Cook over medium heat 1 minute or until cheese melts.
5. Combine 4 egg whites (at room temperature) and cream of tartar; beat until stiff, but not dry. Gently fold into white sauce mixture.
6. Spoon mixture into prepared dish. Bake at 350° for 50 to 60 minutes or until puffed and browned. Serve immediately.

Yield: 8 servings

CHEESE STRATA

Exchanges: 1 Starch, 2 Medium-Fat Meat

Serving Size: ⅙ recipe
Carbohydrate: 20 gm
Protein: 16 gm
Fat: 9 gm

Calories: 227
Fiber: 1 gm
Sodium: 838 mg
Cholesterol: 116 mg

INGREDIENTS:

6 (1-ounce) slices white
  bread, cubed
Vegetable cooking spray
2 cups (8 ounces) shredded
  low-fat process American
  cheese

3 eggs, lightly beaten
2 cups skim milk
¼ teaspoon salt

STEPS IN PREPARATION:

1. Place half of bread cubes in a 1½-quart casserole coated with cooking spray. Layer half of cheese on bread cubes; repeat layers with remaining bread cubes and cheese.
2. Combine eggs, milk, and salt; pour over bread and cheese layers. Cover and chill at least 2 hours.
3. Set casserole in a pan containing ½ inch of hot water. Bake at 325° for 40 to 60 minutes or until a knife inserted in center comes out clean.
4. Cut into 6 equal portions, and serve immediately.

Yield: 6 servings

VEGETARIAN PIZZAS

Exchanges: 2 Starch, 1 Medium-Fat Meat

Serving Size: 1 pizza	**Calories:** 203
Carbohydrate: 32 gm	**Fiber:** 6 gm
Protein: 11 gm	**Sodium:** 495 mg
Fat: 5 gm	**Cholesterol:** 11 mg

INGREDIENTS:

Vegetable cooking spray
½ cup chopped onion
1 clove garlic, minced
4 cups seeded, chopped tomato
2 tablespoons minced fresh basil
3 tablespoons red wine vinegar
2 teaspoons dried oregano
¼ teaspoon pepper
3 (6-inch) whole wheat pita bread rounds

1 cup (4 ounces) shredded low-fat process American cheese
1 medium-size green pepper, chopped
1 small zucchini, thinly sliced
3 ounces fresh mushrooms, thinly sliced
2 tablespoons grated Parmesan cheese

STEPS IN PREPARATION:

1. Coat a large, heavy skillet with cooking spray; place over medium heat until hot. Add onion and garlic, and sauté until tender.
2. Add tomato and next 4 ingredients to skillet. Bring to a boil; reduce heat, and simmer, uncovered, 20 minutes or until reduced by one-third, stirring occasionally.
3. Separate each pita bread into 2 rounds. Place bread rounds on a baking sheet; bake at 450° for 5 minutes or until lightly browned.
4. Spread ¼ cup tomato mixture over each toasted round. Sprinkle shredded cheese evenly over rounds. Arrange chopped pepper, zucchini, and mushrooms over shredded cheese; sprinkle with Parmesan cheese. Bake at 450° for 10 minutes or until cheese melts.

Yield: 6 servings

ZUCCHINI QUICHE

Exchanges: 1 Medium-Fat Meat, 1 Vegetable

Serving Size: 1 wedge	**Calories:** 107
Carbohydrate: 7 gm	**Fiber:** 1 gm
Protein: 8 gm	**Sodium:** 219 mg
Fat: 5 gm	**Cholesterol:** 94 mg

INGREDIENTS:

1 teaspoon cornstarch
¼ teaspoon dried whole
  oregano
1 cup canned stewed
  tomatoes
1½ cups skim milk
1 tablespoon all-purpose
  flour
4 eggs
2 cups shredded zucchini

½ cup (2 ounces) shredded
  Swiss cheese
½ cup (2 ounces) shredded
  low-fat process American
  cheese
¼ cup chopped onion
2 tablespoons grated
  Parmesan cheese
Vegetable cooking spray

STEPS IN PREPARATION:

1. Combine cornstarch and oregano in a small saucepan. Add tomatoes, stirring well; bring to a boil. Reduce heat, and simmer 2 minutes or until thickened. Set aside, and keep warm.
2. Combine milk, flour, and eggs in a large bowl; beat well using a wire whisk. Add zucchini and next 4 ingredients, stirring well.
3. Pour egg mixture into a 9-inch quiche dish coated with cooking spray. Bake at 350° for 1 hour.
4. Spoon tomato mixture over quiche. Cut into 9 wedges, and serve immediately.

Yield: 9 servings

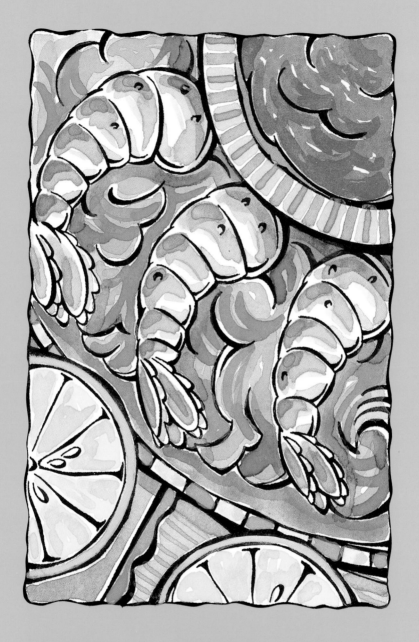

FISH & SHELLFISH

FISH FILLET CASSEROLE

Exchanges: 3 Lean Meat, 1 Vegetable

Serving Size: 3 ounces with sauce
Carbohydrate: 3 gm
Protein: 19 gm
Fat: 4 gm

Calories: 132
Fiber: 0 gm
Sodium: 474 mg
Cholesterol: 52 mg

INGREDIENTS:

1½ pounds fish fillets
Vegetable cooking spray
1 (10¾-ounce) can cream of
   shrimp soup, undiluted
¼ teaspoon hot sauce

½ cup (2 ounces) shredded
   low-fat process American
   cheese
½ teaspoon paprika

STEPS IN PREPARATION:

1. Place fillets, skin side down, in a baking dish coated with cooking spray.
2. Combine soup and hot sauce; spoon over fish.
3. Sprinkle with cheese and paprika; bake at 400° for 35 to 45 minutes or until fish flakes easily when tested with a fork.

Yield: 8 servings

Fresh fish is best when cooked the day you buy it. If you need to keep it overnight, rinse the fish with cold water, pat dry, and wrap it in wax paper. Seal the fish in an airtight plastic bag; place the bag in a bowl of ice cubes, and store in the refrigerator.

BROILED FISH FILLETS

Exchanges: 1 Lean Meat

Serving Size: 1 ounce
Carbohydrate: 1 gm
Protein: 7 gm
Fat: 1gm

Calories: 43
Fiber: 0 gm
Sodium: 146 mg
Cholesterol: 21 mg

INGREDIENTS:

¼ cup commercial no-oil
  Italian dressing
½ teaspoon Worcestershire
  sauce
¼ teaspoon salt

Dash of pepper
¾ pound fish fillets
1 lime, halved
2 green onions, chopped

STEPS IN PREPARATION:

1. Combine first 4 ingredients; add fillets, and marinate in refrigerator 2 hours.
2. Drain fillets, discarding marinade; place in a broiling pan, and broil 8 to 10 minutes or until fish flakes easily when tested with a fork.
3. Squeeze juice of 1 lime half over fillets; broil 1 minute.
4. Remove fillets from oven, and sprinkle with juice of 1 remaining lime half. Sprinkle with green onions before serving.

Yield: 9 servings

CREOLE FISH FILLETS

Exchanges: 1 Lean Meat, 1 Vegetable

Serving Size: ½ cup
Carbohydrate: 6 gm
Protein: 9 gm
Fat: 1 gm

Calories: 70
Fiber: 1 gm
Sodium: 496 mg
Cholesterol: 22 mg

INGREDIENTS:

¾ cup sliced celery
¼ cup chopped onion
1 medium-size green pepper, chopped
1 tablespoon reduced-calorie margarine, melted
1½ cups water
1 (6-ounce) can tomato paste

1 teaspoon salt
¼ teaspoon dried thyme
⅛ teaspoon pepper
Dash of garlic powder
1 bay leaf
2 cups diced cooked fish fillets

STEPS IN PREPARATION:

1. Sauté celery, onion, and green pepper in margarine in a nonstick skillet until vegetables are tender.
2. Add water and next 6 ingredients; simmer 15 minutes, stirring occasionally.
3. Add fillets, and cook until thoroughly heated. Remove and discard bay leaf.
4. Serve fillets over cooked rice (cooked without salt or fat), if desired.

Yield: 8 servings

Note: See the Starch List on page 16 for exchange value of rice.

ORIENTAL BROILED FISH

Exchanges: 1 Lean Meat

Serving Size: 1 ounce	**Calories:** 46
Carbohydrate: 0 gm	**Fiber:** 0 gm
Protein: 7 gm	**Sodium:** 117 mg
Fat: 2 gm	**Cholesterol:** 20 mg

INGREDIENTS:

1 tablespoon vegetable oil
1 tablespoon soy sauce
⅛ teaspoon ground ginger
1 clove garlic, crushed
1 (16-ounce) package frozen
  unbreaded fish fillets,
  thawed

2 tablespoons minced green
  onions

STEPS IN PREPARATION:

1. Combine first 4 ingredients in bottom of a broiling pan. Place fillets in pan, and turn to coat with oil mixture.
2. Cover and marinate in refrigerator at least 1 hour.
3. Broil fillets in marinade 8 to 10 minutes or until fish flakes easily when tested with a fork. Sprinkle with green onions before serving.

Yield: 12 servings

OVEN-FRIED FISH

Exchanges: 2 Lean Meat

Serving Size: 2 ounces	**Calories:** 103
Carbohydrate: 2 gm	**Fiber:** 0 gm
Protein: 16 gm	**Sodium:** 195 mg
Fat: 3 gm	**Cholesterol:** 39 mg

INGREDIENTS:

½ cup crushed corn flakes cereal
½ teaspoon celery salt
⅛ teaspoon onion powder
⅛ teaspoon paprika
Dash of pepper

1 pound catfish or other fish fillets
1 tablespoon plus 1 teaspoon skim milk
Vegetable cooking spray

STEPS IN PREPARATION:

1. Combine first 5 ingredients in a shallow dish.
2. Dip fillets in milk; dredge in cereal mixture.
3. Place fillets in a baking dish coated with cooking spray. Bake at 350° for 25 minutes or until fish is lightly browned and flakes easily when tested with a fork.

Yield: 6 servings

Research shows that fish oils (omega-3 fatty acids) can lower blood pressure and reduce blood clotting. Instead of taking fish oil supplements, add omega-3 fatty acids to your diet by eating salmon, tuna, herring, mackerel, or lake trout twice a week.

BAKED HALIBUT

Exchanges: 3 Lean Meat

Serving Size: 1 steak	**Calories:** 114
Carbohydrate: 1 gm	**Fiber:** trace
Protein: 22 gm	**Sodium:** 220 mg
Fat: 2 gm	**Cholesterol:** 30 mg

INGREDIENTS:

8 (4-ounce) halibut steaks	½ cup water
1 tablespoon Dijon mustard	½ teaspoon chicken-flavored
¼ cup lemon juice	bouillon granules
1 tablespoon vinegar	2 green onions, chopped
½ teaspoon dried oregano	2 tablespoons grated
¼ teaspoon pepper	Parmesan cheese

STEPS IN PREPARATION:

1. Rinse steaks thoroughly in cold water; pat dry with paper towels, and place in a shallow baking dish. Brush steaks evenly with mustard.
2. Combine lemon juice, vinegar, oregano, and pepper. Pour over steaks, and marinate in refrigerator 1 to 2 hours.
3. Combine water and bouillon granules in a small saucepan. Cook over medium heat, stirring constantly, until granules dissolve.
4. Pour broth around steaks in marinade in dish. Top steaks with green onions and cheese. Bake at 375° for 25 minutes or until fish flakes easily when tested with a fork.

Yield: 8 servings

HALIBUT FLORENTINE

Exchanges: 2 Lean Meat, 1 Vegetable

Serving Size: ⅛ recipe	**Calories:** 105
Carbohydrate: 5 gm	**Fiber:** trace
Protein: 14 gm	**Sodium:** 122 mg
Fat: 3 gm	**Cholesterol:** 58 mg

INGREDIENTS:

1 (10-ounce) package frozen chopped spinach
2 tablespoons lemon juice
4 (4-ounce) halibut fillets
1 tablespoon reduced-calorie margarine
2 tablespoons all-purpose flour
1 cup skim milk
1 egg yolk, lightly beaten
¼ cup (1 ounce) shredded reduced-fat Swiss cheese
1 tablespoon grated Parmesan cheese

STEPS IN PREPARATION:

1. Cook spinach according to package directions, omitting salt. Drain well, and place in an 11- x 7- x 2-inch baking dish; sprinkle with lemon juice.
2. Rinse fillets thoroughly in cold water; pat dry with paper towels, and arrange over spinach.
3. Melt margarine in a small saucepan over low heat; add flour, stirring until smooth. Cook, stirring constantly, 1 minute. Gradually add milk; cook over medium heat, stirring constantly, until mixture is thickened and bubbly. Remove from heat, and stir in egg yolk. Add Swiss cheese, and cook over low heat until cheese melts, stirring frequently.
4. Spoon sauce over fillets, and sprinkle with Parmesan cheese. Bake at 350° for 20 minutes or until fish flakes easily when tested with a fork.

Yield: 8 servings

STUFFED FLOUNDER

Exchanges: 1½ Lean Meat, 1 Vegetable

Serving Size: 1 fillet	**Calories:** 100
Carbohydrate: 5 gm	**Fiber:** 1 gm
Protein: 13 gm	**Sodium:** 120 mg
Fat: 2 gm	**Cholesterol:** 36 mg

INGREDIENTS:

4 (3-ounce) flounder fillets
Vegetable cooking spray
½ cup finely chopped onion
1 clove garlic, minced
¼ cup finely chopped celery
¼ cup finely chopped carrot
¼ cup minced sweet red pepper
2 tablespoons chopped fresh parsley, divided

⅛ teaspoon ground thyme
1 tablespoon grated Parmesan cheese
1 tablespoon reduced-calorie mayonnaise
½ teaspoon Dijon mustard
1 tablespoon lemon juice

STEPS IN PREPARATION:

1. Rinse fillets thoroughly in cold water; pat dry with paper towels. Set aside.
2. Coat a medium skillet with cooking spray; place over medium heat until hot. Add onion and garlic; sauté until tender. Add celery, carrot, and pepper; cover and cook over medium-low heat 5 minutes or until vegetables are tender, stirring occasionally. Add 1 tablespoon parsley and thyme.
3. Spoon mixture evenly into centers of fillets; roll up lengthwise, and secure with wooden picks. Place rolls, seam side down, in a shallow baking dish coated with cooking spray.
4. Combine cheese, mayonnaise, and mustard; spread mixture evenly over rolls, and sprinkle with lemon juice. Bake at 400° for 20 minutes or until fish is lightly browned and flakes easily when tested with a fork. Sprinkle with remaining 1 tablespoon parsley. Serve immediately.

Yield: 4 servings

CURRIED FLOUNDER

Exchanges: 2 Lean Meat

Serving Size: 1 fillet	**Calories:** 87
Carbohydrate: 2 gm	**Fiber:** trace
Protein: 15 gm	**Sodium:** 82 mg
Fat: 2 gm	**Cholesterol:** 42 mg

INGREDIENTS:

8 (3-ounce) flounder fillets
2 green onions, minced
2 small cloves garlic, minced
⅛ teaspoon curry powder
⅛ teaspoon red pepper

2 tablespoons all-purpose flour
1 tablespoon reduced-calorie margarine

STEPS IN PREPARATION:

1. Rinse fillets thoroughly in cold water; pat dry with paper towels, and place in a shallow baking dish.
2. Combine green onions and next 3 ingredients; rub over fillets. Cover and chill 1 hour.
3. Remove fillets from baking dish, and coat with flour.
4. Melt margarine in baking dish in a 350° oven; add fillets, turning once. Bake for 8 to 10 minutes or until fish flakes easily when tested with a fork.

Yield: 8 servings

Cooking time is critical with fish because the flesh is so delicate. Perfectly cooked fish will be moist and tender; overcooked fish will be dry and tough. When fish is cooked to perfection, the translucent flesh turns opaque (or solid) in appearance, and it flakes easily with a fork.

BAKED SALMON

Exchanges: 2 Lean Meat

Serving Size: 1 steak	**Calories:** 103
Carbohydrate: 1 gm	**Fiber:** trace
Protein: 15 gm	**Sodium:** 44 mg
Fat: 4 gm	**Cholesterol:** 46 mg

INGREDIENTS:

4 (2½-ounce) salmon steaks
Vegetable cooking spray
2 tablespoons lemon juice
½ teaspoon dried dillweed

½ teaspoon dried parsley
  flakes
½ teaspoon pepper

STEPS IN PREPARATION:

1. Rinse steaks thoroughly in cold water; pat dry with paper towels.
2. Place steaks in a shallow pan coated with cooking spray; brush with lemon juice. Sprinkle evenly with dillweed, parsley, and pepper.
3. Bake at 350° for 25 to 35 minutes or until fish flakes easily when tested with a fork.

Yield: 4 servings

SALMON CROQUETTES

Exchanges: 1 Starch, 3 Lean Meat

Serving Size: 1 croquette	**Calories:** 192
Carbohydrate: 12 gm	**Fiber:** 0 gm
Protein: 21 gm	**Sodium:** 274 mg
Fat: 6 gm	**Cholesterol:** 51 mg

INGREDIENTS:

1 (16-ounce) can no-salt-added salmon
⅔ cup skim milk
2 teaspoons reduced-calorie margarine
2 tablespoons minced onion
¼ cup all-purpose flour
¾ teaspoon hot sauce
¼ teaspoon salt
Dash of pepper
1 tablespoon lemon juice
1 cup crushed corn flakes cereal, divided
5 lemon wedges (optional)

STEPS IN PREPARATION:

1. Drain salmon, reserving liquid; add milk to salmon liquid.
2. Melt margarine in a nonstick skillet; add onion, and sauté until tender. Add flour and next 3 ingredients to onion mixture; stir well. Add milk mixture, and cook over low heat, stirring constantly, until thickened.
3. Flake salmon; add salmon and lemon juice to sauce. Stir in ½ cup cereal.
4. Cover and chill 1 hour.
5. Divide mixture into ½-cup portions, and shape into cones; roll cones in remaining ½ cup cereal, coating well.
6. Place on a nonstick baking sheet, and bake at 400° for 20 to 25 minutes or until lightly browned. Garnish with lemon wedges, if desired.

Yield: 5 servings

LEMON-BAKED SOLE

Exchanges: 2 Lean Meat

Serving Size: 1 fillet	**Calories:** 98
Carbohydrate: 3 gm	**Fiber:** trace
Protein: 16 gm	**Sodium:** 91 mg
Fat: 2 gm	**Cholesterol:** 43 mg

INGREDIENTS:

4 (4-ounce) sole fillets
2 teaspoons reduced-calorie margarine, melted
2 teaspoons lemon juice
2 tablespoons all-purpose flour
2 teaspoons chopped fresh parsley
⅛ teaspoon pepper
⅛ teaspoon paprika
Lemon wedges (optional)
Fresh parsley sprigs (optional)

STEPS IN PREPARATION:

1. Rinse fillets thoroughly in cold water; pat dry with paper towels, and set aside.
2. Combine margarine and lemon juice in a small bowl. Combine flour, chopped parsley, and pepper in a shallow dish. Dip fillets in margarine mixture, and dredge in flour mixture.
3. Transfer fillets to a nonstick baking sheet, and drizzle remaining margarine mixture over fillets. Sprinkle with paprika.
4. Bake at 375° for 15 to 20 minutes or until fish is golden and flakes easily when tested with a fork. If desired, garnish with lemon wedges and parsley sprigs.

Yield: 4 servings

VEGETABLE-TOPPED SNAPPER

Exchanges: 3 Lean Meat, 1 Vegetable

Serving Size: 1 fillet
Carbohydrate: 6 gm
Protein: 23 gm
Fat: 5 gm

Calories: 162
Fiber: 1 gm
Sodium: 403 mg
Cholesterol: 61 mg

INGREDIENTS:

6 (4-ounce) snapper fillets
½ teaspoon dried tarragon
¼ teaspoon salt
¼ teaspoon pepper
Vegetable cooking spray
1 medium onion, chopped
¼ pound fresh mushrooms, sliced

3 tablespoons reduced-calorie margarine, melted
1 medium tomato, seeded and chopped
¼ cup reduced-calorie ketchup
2 tablespoons grated Parmesan cheese

STEPS IN PREPARATION:

1. Rinse fillets thoroughly in cold water; pat dry with paper towels.
2. Sprinkle fillets with tarragon, salt, and pepper, and place in a 13- x 9- x 2-inch baking dish coated with cooking spray. Bake, uncovered, at 500° for 10 to 12 minutes or until fish flakes easily when tested with a fork.
3. Sauté onion and mushrooms in margarine in a large skillet until vegetables are tender. Remove from heat, and stir in tomato and ketchup.
4. Remove fillets from oven; drain. Spoon onion mixture evenly over fillets, and sprinkle with cheese. Broil 3 inches from heat until cheese melts. Serve immediately.

Yield: 6 servings

TUNA CREOLE

Exchanges: 2 Lean Meat, 2 Vegetable

Serving Size: 1 cup	**Calories:** 136
Carbohydrate: 9 gm	**Fiber:** 2 gm
Protein: 18 gm	**Sodium:** 679 mg
Fat: 3 gm	**Cholesterol:** 10 mg

INGREDIENTS:

1 cup chopped onion
2 tablespoons chopped green pepper
2 tablespoons reduced-calorie margarine, melted
2 tablespoons all-purpose flour
1 (14½-ounce) can tomatoes
¼ cup sliced stuffed olives
½ teaspoon dried oregano
½ teaspoon salt
⅛ teaspoon pepper
⅛ teaspoon ground allspice
2 (6½-ounce) cans tuna in water

STEPS IN PREPARATION:

1. Sauté onion and green pepper in margarine in a nonstick skillet until vegetables are tender.
2. Add flour; stirring well. Add tomatoes and next 5 ingredients; cook, stirring constantly, until thickened.
3. Drain and flake tuna; stir into tomato mixture.
4. Serve over cooked rice or noodles (cooked without salt or fat), if desired.

Yield: 6 servings

Note: See the Starch List on page 16 for exchange values of rice and noodles.

TUNA SALAD

Exchanges: 2 Lean Meat

Serving Size: ½ cup
Carbohydrate: 2 gm
Protein: 15 gm
Fat: 2 gm

Calories: 95
Fiber: 0 gm
Sodium: 283 mg
Cholesterol: 101 mg

INGREDIENTS:

1 (6½-ounce) can tuna in
  water, drained and flaked
2 hard-cooked eggs, chopped
¼ cup chopped celery

2 tablespoons nonfat
  mayonnaise
Lettuce leaves (optional)

STEPS IN PREPARATION:

1. Combine first 4 ingredients in a small bowl. Cover and chill.
2. Serve on lettuce leaves, if desired.

Yield: 4 servings

Canned tuna is available in the following forms:
tuna packed in oil or spring water, chunk or solid
pack, and light tuna or albacore tuna. Tuna packed
in water contains 36 calories per ounce versus 82
calories for the same amount of tuna packed in oil.

SPICY TUNA PASTA TOSS

Exchanges: 1 Starch, 2 Lean Meat, 2 Vegetable

Serving Size: 1 cup
Carbohydrate: 25 gm
Protein: 17 gm
Fat: 7 gm

Calories: 236
Fiber: 1 gm
Sodium: 341 mg
Cholesterol: 26 mg

INGREDIENTS:

6 ounces tri-colored corkscrew pasta, uncooked
2 (6⅛-ounce) cans chunk white tuna in spring water, drained
½ cup sweet yellow pepper strips
½ cup quartered cherry tomatoes
¼ cup diced celery
¾ cup no-salt-added commercial salsa
½ cup reduced-calorie mayonnaise
½ teaspoon ground red pepper
Curly leaf lettuce leaves (optional)
2 tablespoons sliced green onions

STEPS IN PREPARATION:

1. Cook pasta according to package directions, omitting salt and fat. Drain; rinse under cold water, and drain. Combine pasta, tuna, and next 3 ingredients.
2. Combine salsa, mayonnaise, and red pepper in a small bowl. Add to pasta mixture; toss. Cover and chill.
3. Serve in a lettuce-lined bowl, if desired; sprinkle with green onions.

Yield: 6 servings

STIR-FRIED TUNA

Exchanges: 1 Starch, 2 Lean Meat

Serving Size: ¾ cup
Carbohydrate: 12 gm
Protein: 18 gm
Fat: trace

Calories: 126
Fiber: 2 gm
Sodium: 522 mg
Cholesterol: 10 mg

INGREDIENTS:

Vegetable cooking spray
1 medium-size sweet red or green pepper, coarsely chopped
8 green onions, cut into ½-inch pieces
1 clove garlic, minced
1 cup diagonally sliced celery
5 ounces fresh snow pea pods
2 ounces fresh mushrooms, sliced
1 (8-ounce) can sliced water chestnuts, drained
1 tablespoon cornstarch
3 tablespoons reduced-sodium soy sauce
3 tablespoons water
1 tablespoon vinegar
¼ teaspoon ground ginger
2 (6½-ounce) cans tuna in water, drained and flaked

STEPS IN PREPARATION:

1. Coat a wok or large heavy skillet with cooking spray; heat at medium-high (375°) for 2 minutes. Add pepper, green onions, and garlic; stir-fry 15 seconds. Add celery and next 3 ingredients; stir-fry 1 minute or until vegetables are crisp-tender.
2. Combine cornstarch and next 4 ingredients, stirring until cornstarch dissolves; add to wok. Cook over medium-high heat until sauce is slightly thickened, stirring frequently. Add tuna, stirring to coat well.
3. Serve over cooked rice (cooked without salt or fat), if desired.

Yield: 6 servings

Note: See the Starch List on page 16 for exchange value of rice.

TUNA PILAF

Exchanges: 1 Starch, 1 Lean Meat, 1 Vegetable

Serving Size: ½ cup
Carbohydrate: 18 gm
Protein: 14 gm
Fat: 1 gm

Calories: 275
Fiber: 2 gm
Sodium: 454 mg
Cholesterol: 13 mg

INGREDIENTS:

2 green onions, chopped
1 teaspoon reduced-calorie margarine, melted
2½ cups water
1 cup long-grain rice, uncooked
1 (10-ounce) package frozen mixed Oriental vegetables, thawed
1 (10-ounce) can tuna in water, drained and broken into chunks
1 tablespoon reduced-sodium soy sauce

STEPS IN PREPARATION:

1. Sauté onions in margarine in a large saucepan until onions are tender.
2. Add water; bring to a boil. Stir in rice; cover, reduce heat, and simmer 20 to 25 minutes or until rice is tender and liquid is absorbed.
3. Add mixed vegetables. Cook over low heat 5 minutes or until vegetables are tender.
4. Add tuna and soy sauce; stir. Serve warm.

Yield: 8 servings

SHRIMP SALAD

Exchanges: 2 Lean Meat, 1 Vegetable

Serving Size: ⅓ cup
Carbohydrate: 4 gm
Protein: 17 gm
Fat: 1 gm

Calories: 96
Fiber: 0 gm
Sodium: 393 mg
Cholesterol: 161 mg

INGREDIENTS:

3 cups water
1 pound unpeeled medium-size fresh shrimp
¼ cup nonfat mayonnaise
¾ teaspoon diced pimiento
¾ teaspoon lemon juice

½ teaspoon prepared mustard
⅛ teaspoon ground white pepper
⅛ teaspoon chopped parsley
⅓ cup finely chopped celery

STEPS IN PREPARATION:

1. Bring 3 cups water to a boil in a medium saucepan. Add shrimp; cook 5 minutes or until shrimp turns pink. Drain well; cool. Peel and devein shrimp; chop.
2. Combine mayonnaise and next 5 ingredients; stir well.
3. Add shrimp and celery to mayonnaise mixture. Cover and chill.

Yield: 4 servings

The key to lowering blood cholesterol is to cut down on high-cholesterol foods and foods that are high in saturated fat.

Although shrimp is higher in cholesterol than some other types of shellfish, it is very low in saturated fat. A 3-ounce portion of shrimp contains 166 milligrams of cholesterol, so you can include shrimp in your diet and still stay below the American Heart Association's recommendation of no more than 300 milligrams of cholesterol per day.

SHRIMP-MACARONI SALAD

Exchanges: ½ Starch, 1 Lean Meat

Serving Size: ¾ cup	**Calories:** 100
Carbohydrate: 11 gm	**Fiber:** 1 gm
Protein: 6 gm	**Sodium:** 212 mg
Fat: 4 gm	**Cholesterol:** 42 mg

INGREDIENTS:

¾ cup uncooked shell macaroni
3 cups water
¾ pound medium-size fresh shrimp, peeled and deveined
1 cup chopped cauliflower
1 cup sliced celery
½ cup commercial low-calorie French dressing
¼ cup chopped fresh parsley
¼ cup chopped sweet pickle
¼ cup reduced-calorie mayonnaise
1 tablespoon lemon juice
1 teaspoon grated onion
½ teaspoon celery seeds
¼ teaspoon pepper

STEPS IN PREPARATION:

1. Cook macaroni according to package directions, omitting salt and fat. Drain and set aside.
2. Bring 3 cups water to a boil in a medium saucepan. Add shrimp; cook 3 to 5 minutes or until shrimp turns pink. Drain well.
3. Combine macaroni, shrimp, cauliflower, and remaining ingredients; toss gently to combine. Cover and chill at least 8 hours.

Yield: 12 servings

SHRIMP SCAMPI

Exchanges: 2 Lean Meat

Serving Size: ¼ recipe
Carbohydrate: 5 gm
Protein: 15 gm
Fat: 1 gm

Calories: 93
Fiber: 0 gm
Sodium: 693 mg
Cholesterol: 125 mg

INGREDIENTS:

3 cups water
¾ pound medium-size fresh shrimp, peeled and deveined
1½ cups fat-free chicken broth
½ cup dry butter substitute
1½ tablespoons lemon juice
½ teaspoon salt
½ teaspoon garlic powder
½ teaspoon dried parsley flakes
¼ teaspoon dried oregano leaves
¼ teaspoon dried basil
⅛ teaspoon ground red pepper
1 tablespoon cornstarch

STEPS IN PREPARATION:

1. Bring 3 cups water to a boil in a medium saucepan. Add shrimp; cook 3 minutes. Drain well, and set aside.
2. Combine broth and next 8 ingredients in a medium saucepan. Bring to a boil, and add shrimp. Add cornstarch; cook, stirring constantly, until thickened.
3. Serve over cooked rice (cooked without salt or fat), if desired.

Yield: 4 servings

Note: See the Starch List on page 16 for exchange value of rice.

SHRIMP AND CHICKEN CREOLE

Exchanges: 3 Lean Meat, 2 Vegetable

Serving Size: 1 cup
Carbohydrate: 9 gm
Protein: 20 gm
Fat: 3 gm

Calories: 140
Fiber: 2 gm
Sodium: 326 mg
Cholesterol: 122 mg

INGREDIENTS:

1 cup chopped green pepper
¾ cup chopped onion
1 teaspoon vegetable oil
2 cups peeled, diced tomato
½ teaspoon salt
½ teaspoon garlic powder
½ teaspoon chili powder
¼ teaspoon ground red pepper

⅛ teaspoon black pepper
¾ pound small fresh shrimp, peeled and deveined
1 cup chopped cooked chicken (skinned before cooking and cooked without salt)

STEPS IN PREPARATION:

1. Sauté green pepper and onion in oil in a skillet until vegetables are tender.
2. Stir in tomato and next 5 ingredients. Bring to a boil. Reduce heat, and simmer, uncovered, 20 to 30 minutes or until thickened.
3. Stir in shrimp and chicken (mixture will thin when shrimp is added). Return to a boil; reduce heat, and cook 1 to 2 minutes or until shrimp turns pink.
4. Serve over cooked rice (cooked without salt or fat), if desired.

Yield: 6 servings

Note: See the Starch List on page 16 for exchange value of rice.

CURRY-SHRIMP CREOLE

Exchanges: 1 Lean Meat, 1½ Vegetable

Serving Size: ½ cup	**Calories:** 80
Carbohydrate: 8 gm	**Fiber:** 1 gm
Protein: 8 gm	**Sodium:** 393 mg
Fat: 2 gm	**Cholesterol:** 61 mg

INGREDIENTS:

2 medium onions, chopped
1 medium-size green pepper, cut into 1-inch pieces
1 stalk celery, sliced
1 clove garlic, minced
1 tablespoon vegetable oil
1 (16-ounce) can whole tomatoes, undrained and chopped
¼ cup minced fresh parsley
¼ cup reduced-calorie ketchup
1 teaspoon lemon juice
½ teaspoon salt
½ teaspoon hot sauce
¼ teaspoon curry powder
¼ teaspoon dried thyme
¾ pound medium-size fresh shrimp, peeled and deveined

STEPS IN PREPARATION:

1. Sauté first 4 ingredients in oil in a large skillet until vegetables are crisp-tender.
2. Stir in tomato and next 7 ingredients. Cover and bring to a boil. Reduce heat, and simmer 30 minutes.
3. Add shrimp. Cover and simmer 5 minutes or until shrimp turns pink.
4. Serve over cooked rice (cooked without salt or fat), if desired.

Yield: 8 servings

Note: See the Starch List on page 16 for exchange value of rice.

SHRIMP STIR-FRY

Exchanges: 2 Lean Meat, 1 Vegetable

Serving Size: ¾ cup
Carbohydrate: 7 gm
Protein: 14 gm
Fat: 3 gm

Calories: 112
Fiber: 2 gm
Sodium: 362 mg
Cholesterol: 107 mg

INGREDIENTS:

1 tablespoon vegetable oil
1 medium onion, thinly sliced
½ cup thinly sliced celery
1 pound medium-size fresh shrimp, peeled and deveined
6 ounces fresh mushrooms, sliced
½ teaspoon minced garlic

1 cup shredded fresh spinach
4 ounces frozen English peas, thawed
1 teaspoon cornstarch
¼ cup water
2 tablespoons reduced-sodium soy sauce

STEPS IN PREPARATION:

1. Coat a wok or large heavy skillet with oil. Heat at medium-high (375°) 2 minutes.
2. Add onion and celery to wok; stir-fry 3 minutes. Add shrimp, mushrooms, and garlic; stir-fry 1 minute or until shrimp turns pink. Add spinach and English peas; stir-fry 30 seconds.
3. Combine cornstarch, water, and soy sauce, stirring until cornstarch dissolves; add to shrimp mixture in wok. Cook, stirring constantly, over medium-high heat until mixture thickens.
4. Serve over hot cooked brown rice (cooked without salt or fat), if desired.

Yield: 6 servings

Note: See the Starch List on page 16 for exchange value of brown rice.

SEAFOOD NEWBURG

Exchanges: ½ Starch, 3 Lean Meat

Serving Size: ¾ cup	**Calories:** 155
Carbohydrate: 8 gm	**Fiber:** 0 gm
Protein: 26 gm	**Sodium:** 565 mg
Fat: 2 gm	**Cholesterol:** 126 mg

INGREDIENTS:

3 cups fat-free chicken broth
1 pound medium-size fresh shrimp, peeled and deveined
¾ pound scallops
½ cup dry butter substitute
½ teaspoon garlic powder
½ teaspoon dried parsley flakes

¼ teaspoon salt
¼ teaspoon ground white pepper
¼ teaspoon dried thyme
¼ teaspoon dried sage
3 tablespoons cornstarch
3 tablespoons water
2 tablespoons lemon juice

STEPS IN PREPARATION:

1. Bring broth to a boil in a medium saucepan. Add shrimp and scallops; cook 3 to 5 minutes or until shrimp turns pink. Remove seafood from broth; set seafood aside.
2. Add butter substitute and next 6 ingredients to broth; bring to a boil.
3. Combine cornstarch and water; add to chicken broth mixture. Reduce heat, and simmer 5 minutes. Add lemon juice to broth mixture; add shrimp and scallops, and stir.
4. Serve over cooked rice (cooked without salt or fat), if desired.

Yield: 6 servings

Note: See the Starch List on page 16 for exchange value of rice.

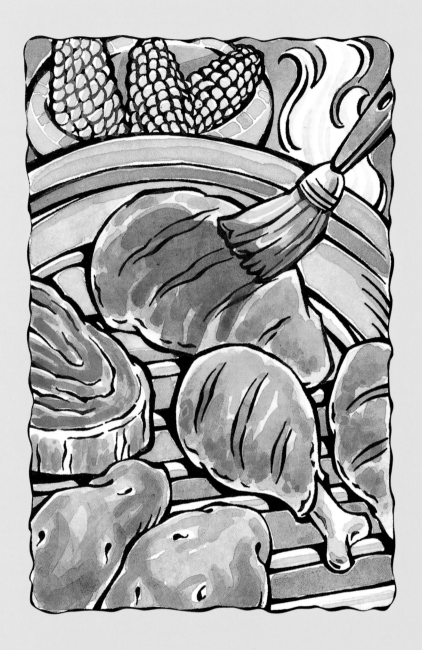

MEATS

BEEFY CHILI

Exchanges: 1 Starch, 1 Medium-Fat Meat

Serving Size: ½ cup
Carbohydrate: 11 gm
Protein: 9 gm
Fat: 4 gm

Calories: 118
Fiber: 4 gm
Sodium: 295 mg
Cholesterol: 16 mg

INGREDIENTS:

1 pound lean ground beef
½ cup chopped onion
1 tablespoon chili powder
1 teaspoon salt
1 (16-ounce) can crushed
   tomatoes, undrained

1 (15-ounce) can kidney
   beans, undrained
3 cups water

STEPS IN PREPARATION:

1. Combine first 4 ingredients in a nonstick skillet. Cook over medium heat until meat is browned, stirring until meat crumbles. Drain and pat dry with paper towels.
2. Combine tomato and beans in a saucepan. Add water.
3. Add meat mixture to saucepan. Bring to a boil; reduce heat, and simmer, uncovered, 1 hour.

Yield: 16 servings

GROUND BEEF PIE

Exchanges: 1 Starch, 2 Medium-Fat Meat

Serving Size: ⅛ recipe
Carbohydrate: 18 gm
Protein: 17 gm
Fat: 8 gm

Calories: 216
Fiber: 6 gm
Sodium: 783 mg
Cholesterol: 33 mg

INGREDIENTS:

1 pound lean ground beef
1 small onion, finely chopped
1 teaspoon salt
½ teaspoon chili powder
⅛ teaspoon pepper
Vegetable cooking spray

1 cup tomato juice
1 (16-ounce) can green beans,
   drained
2½ cups mashed potatoes
   (cooked without salt or fat)
¼ teaspoon paprika

STEPS IN PREPARATION:

1. Combine first 5 ingredients in a nonstick skillet. Cook over medium heat until meat is browned, stirring until meat crumbles. Drain and pat dry with paper towels.
2. Place meat mixture in a 2-quart casserole coated with cooking spray. Pour tomato juice over meat mixture.
3. Arrange beans over meat mixture.
4. Spoon mashed potatoes over beans. Sprinkle with paprika. Bake at 350° for 35 to 40 minutes or until golden.

Yield: 8 servings

ENCHILADA PIE

Exchanges: 2 Medium-Fat Meat, 1 Vegetable

Serving Size: ½ cup
Carbohydrate: 8 gm
Protein: 14 gm
Fat: 10 gm

Calories: 180
Fiber: 1 gm
Sodium: 356 mg
Cholesterol: 38 mg

INGREDIENTS:

1 pound ground chuck
½ cup chopped onion
1 (4-ounce) can tomato sauce
1 teaspoon chili powder
½ teaspoon ground cumin
¼ teaspoon salt
¼ teaspoon pepper

4 (6-inch) corn tortillas
¾ cup (3 ounces) shredded
   low-fat process American
   cheese
Vegetable cooking spray
½ cup water

STEPS IN PREPARATION:

1. Cook ground chuck and onion in a large nonstick skillet over medium heat until browned, stirring until meat crumbles. Drain and pat dry with paper towels.
2. Return meat to skillet; stir in tomato sauce and next 4 ingredients. Cook over medium heat, stirring constantly, until thoroughly heated.
3. Layer tortillas, meat sauce, and cheese in a 2-quart casserole coated with cooking spray; pour water over top. Cover and bake at 400° for 20 minutes. Serve warm.

Yield: 8 servings

SAVORY HASH

Exchanges: 2 Medium-Fat Meat, 1 Vegetable

Serving Size: ½ cup	**Calories:** 214
Carbohydrate: 13 gm	**Fiber:** 2 gm
Protein: 16 gm	**Sodium:** 477 mg
Fat: 11 gm	**Cholesterol:** 43 mg

INGREDIENTS:

1 pound lean ground beef
½ cup finely chopped celery
½ cup finely chopped onion
¼ cup finely chopped green pepper
2 cups chopped tomato

½ cup cooked long-grain rice (cooked without salt or fat)
1 teaspoon chili powder
1 teaspoon salt
¼ teaspoon pepper

STEPS IN PREPARATION:

1. Cook first 4 ingredients in a nonstick skillet over medium heat until meat is browned, stirring until meat crumbles. Drain and pat dry with paper towels.
2. Return meat mixture to skillet; add tomato and remaining ingredients. Cover and cook over low heat 45 minutes, adding water occasionally to keep meat from sticking to skillet.

Yield: 6 servings

For maximum reduction of fat, use ultra-lean ground beef. Consider this difference: a 3-ounce cooked portion of ultra-lean ground beef contains 7 grams of fat; 3 ounces of cooked lean ground beef contain about 14 grams of fat.

ITALIAN SPAGHETTI

Exchanges: 1 Starch, 1 Medium-Fat Meat, 1 Vegetable

Serving Size: 1 cup	**Calories:** 250
Carbohydrate: 28 gm	**Fiber:** 3 gm
Protein: 15 gm	**Sodium:** 302 mg
Fat: 9 gm	**Cholesterol:** 32 mg

INGREDIENTS:

½ pound lean ground beef
½ small onion, chopped
⅔ cup water
½ cup chopped tomato
⅓ cup tomato paste
2½ teaspoons Italian seasoning

½ teaspoon onion powder
¼ teaspoon garlic powder
¼ teaspoon dried oregano
⅛ teaspoon pepper
1 small bay leaf
2 cups cooked spaghetti (cooked without salt or fat)

STEPS IN PREPARATION:

1. Cook ground beef and onion in a nonstick skillet over medium heat until meat is browned, stirring until meat crumbles. Drain and pat dry with paper towels.
2. Return meat mixture to skillet; add water and next 8 ingredients. Bring to a boil; reduce heat, and simmer, covered, 1 hour. Add more water if needed.
3. To serve, remove and discard bay leaf. Spoon ½ cup sauce over ½ cup cooked spaghetti.

Yield: 4 servings

STUFFED PEPPERS

Exchanges: 2 Starch, 1½ Medium-Fat Meat

Serving Size: 1 stuffed pepper
Carbohydrate: 34 gm
Protein: 15 gm
Fat: 9 gm

Calories: 273
Fiber: 3 gm
Sodium: 908 mg
Cholesterol: 33 mg

INGREDIENTS:

4 medium-size green peppers
½ pound lean ground beef
½ cup chopped onion
1 cup canned tomatoes, drained
1 cup cooked long-grain rice (cooked without salt or fat)
1 tablespoon Worcestershire sauce
½ teaspoon Italian seasoning
¼ teaspoon salt
Dash of pepper
¼ cup soft breadcrumbs
Vegetable cooking spray
1 cup canned tomato sauce

STEPS IN PREPARATION:

1. Slice off stem end of peppers; remove and discard seeds and membranes. Blanch peppers 5 to 10 minutes in boiling water. Drain.
2. Cook ground beef and onion in a nonstick skillet over medium heat until meat is browned, stirring until meat crumbles. Drain and pat dry with paper towels.
3. Return meat mixture to skillet. Add tomatoes; cook until liquid evaporates.
4. Remove from heat; stir in rice and next 4 ingredients.
5. Spoon ½-cup portions of rice mixture into peppers; sprinkle evenly with breadcrumbs. Place peppers in a baking dish coated with cooking spray. Bake at 350° for 20 minutes or until lightly browned.
6. Heat tomato sauce; spoon ¼ cup sauce over each pepper.

Yield: 4 servings

GREEN PEPPER CASSEROLE

Exchanges: 1 Medium-Fat Meat, 1 Vegetable

Serving Size: ⅔ cup	**Calories:** 117
Carbohydrate: 6 gm	**Fiber:** 2 gm
Protein: 9 gm	**Sodium:** 30 mg
Fat: 6 gm	**Cholesterol:** 53 mg

INGREDIENTS:

½ pound ground chuck
Vegetable cooking spray
3 medium-size green peppers, finely chopped
2 medium onions, finely chopped
2 tablespoons chopped green onions

1 egg, lightly beaten
2 tablespoons minced fresh parsley
½ teaspoon dried thyme
¼ teaspoon pepper
¼ teaspoon garlic powder
⅛ teaspoon ground cloves
⅛ teaspoon ground allspice

STEPS IN PREPARATION:

1. Cook ground chuck in a Dutch oven over medium heat until browned, stirring until meat crumbles. Drain and pat dry with paper towels. Set meat aside.
2. Wipe Dutch oven with a paper towel; coat with cooking spray, and place over low heat until hot.
3. Add green pepper, onion, and green onions; sauté 5 minutes or until vegetables are tender. Return meat to Dutch oven. Add egg and remaining ingredients, stirring well.
4. Spoon mixture into a shallow 2-quart casserole coated with cooking spray. Bake at 375° for 20 minutes or until set.

Yield: 6 servings

CREOLE MEAT LOAF

Exchanges: 2 Medium-Fat Meat, 2 Vegetable

Serving Size: 1 slice	**Calories:** 206
Carbohydrate: 8 gm	**Fiber:** 1 gm
Protein: 17 gm	**Sodium:** 452 mg
Fat: 12 gm	**Cholesterol:** 75 mg

INGREDIENTS:

1 pound ground chuck
½ cup chopped onion
½ cup skim milk
½ teaspoon dry mustard
½ teaspoon salt
1 egg, lightly beaten
Vegetable cooking spray
½ cup chopped green pepper

3 tablespoons chopped onion
1½ cups tomato juice
¾ cup sliced fresh
  mushrooms
2 tablespoons water
1 teaspoon cornstarch
¼ teaspoon dried thyme

STEPS IN PREPARATION:

1. Combine first 6 ingredients, stirring well. Shape into a loaf, and place in an 8½- x 4½- x 3-inch loafpan coated with cooking spray. Bake at 350° for 1 hour. Cool in pan 10 minutes.
2. Coat a medium skillet with cooking spray; place over low heat until hot. Add green pepper and 3 tablespoons onion; sauté 2 to 3 minutes or until tender.
3. Remove from heat; add tomato juice and mushrooms.
4. Combine water, cornstarch, and thyme, stirring to blend; add to skillet, and bring to a boil. Boil, stirring constantly, 1 minute or until thickened and bubbly.
5. Invert meat loaf onto a serving platter, and spoon tomato juice mixture over meat loaf. To serve, cut meat loaf into 6 slices.

Yield: 6 servings

LASAGNA

Exchanges: 1 Starch, 2 Medium-Fat Meat

Serving Size: 1/12 recipe	**Calories:** 205
Carbohydrate: 17 gm	**Fiber:** 2 gm
Protein: 16 gm	**Sodium:** 333 mg
Fat: 8 gm	**Cholesterol:** 45 mg

INGREDIENTS:

1 pound ground chuck
½ cup water
1 (16-ounce) can stewed tomatoes, undrained
2 teaspoons dried Italian seasoning
1 clove garlic, minced
1 (8-ounce) package whole wheat lasagna noodles
1 (10-ounce) package frozen chopped spinach

1 cup 1% low-fat cottage cheese
2 tablespoons grated Parmesan cheese
1 tablespoon dried parsley flakes
1 teaspoon dried oregano
Vegetable cooking spray
1 cup (4 ounces) shredded low-fat process American cheese

STEPS IN PREPARATION:

1. Cook ground chuck in a medium skillet over medium heat until browned, stirring until meat crumbles. Drain and pat dry with paper towels. Wipe skillet with a paper towel.
2. Return meat to skillet, and stir in water and next 3 ingredients. Cover and bring to a boil. Reduce heat, and simmer 20 minutes.
3. Cook noodles according to package directions, omitting salt and fat. Drain well, and set aside.
4. Cook spinach according to package directions, omitting salt and fat. Drain well, and squeeze excess moisture from spinach. Combine spinach and next 4 ingredients, stirring well.
5. Place half of noodles in a 13- x 9- x 2-inch baking dish coated with cooking spray. Top with half of spinach mixture, half of American cheese, and half of meat mixture.
6. Repeat layers with remaining noodles, spinach mixture, American cheese, and meat mixture. Bake at 350° for 30 minutes. Let stand 10 minutes before serving.

Yield: 12 servings

SIX-LAYER BEEF DINNER

Exchanges: 1 Starch, 1½ Medium-Fat Meat

Serving Size: ¾ cup
Carbohydrate: 19 gm
Protein: 12 gm
Fat: 8 gm

Calories: 202
Fiber: 3 gm
Sodium: 139 mg
Cholesterol: 32 mg

INGREDIENTS:

1 pound ground chuck
4 medium-size round red potatoes, peeled and cut into ¼-inch slices
2 large carrots, scraped and cut into ¼-inch slices
1 large onion, cut into ¼-inch slices

1 medium-size green pepper, cut into ¼-inch slices
1 (16-ounce) can whole tomatoes, undrained and chopped
¼ teaspoon pepper
⅛ teaspoon dried basil

STEPS IN PREPARATION:

1. Cook ground chuck in a large ovenproof skillet over medium heat until meat is browned, stirring until meat crumbles. Drain and pat dry with paper towels. Wipe skillet with a paper towel.
2. Return meat to skillet; layer potato and next 4 ingredients over meat. Sprinkle with ¼ teaspoon pepper and basil. Cover and bake at 350° for 45 minutes. Serve warm.

Yield: 8 servings

You don't have to give up beef if you are trying to lower your blood cholesterol. The American Heart Association guidelines allow up to 6 ounces of lean cooked meat, fish, or poultry each day. A 3-ounce serving of lean beef contains an acceptable level of saturated fat and dietary cholesterol when all visible fat is trimmed.

BEEF AND VEGETABLE KABOBS

Exchanges: 3 Lean Meat, 4 Vegetable

Serving Size: 2 kabobs
Carbohydrate: 21 gm
Protein: 31 gm
Fat: 10 gm

Calories: 290
Fiber: 4 gm
Sodium: 80 mg
Cholesterol: 80 mg

INGREDIENTS:

1 pound lean boneless beef sirloin steak
¼ cup dry red wine
¼ cup reduced-calorie maple syrup
2 tablespoons red wine vinegar
1 teaspoon minced garlic
1 teaspoon curry powder
½ teaspoon pepper
1½ teaspoons olive oil

4 small onions, quartered
2 small sweet red peppers, seeded and cut into 1-inch pieces
2 medium zucchini, each cut into 4 pieces
2 medium-size yellow squash, each cut into 4 pieces
8 medium-size fresh mushrooms
Vegetable cooking spray

STEPS IN PREPARATION:

1. Trim fat from steak; cut steak into 1-inch pieces. Place steak in a heavy-duty, zip-top plastic bag. Combine wine and next 6 ingredients in a small bowl, stirring well. Pour over steak. Seal bag, and shake until steak is well coated. Marinate in refrigerator at least 8 hours, turning bag occasionally.
2. Remove steak from marinade, reserving marinade. Place marinade in a small saucepan; bring to a boil. Reduce heat, and simmer 2 minutes.
3. Thread steak, onion, and next 4 ingredients alternately onto 8 (10-inch) skewers. Coat grill rack with cooking spray; place on grill over medium-hot coals (350° to 400°). Place kabobs on rack, and grill, covered, 12 to 14 minutes or to desired degree of doneness, turning and basting often with marinade.

Yield: 4 servings

GINGERED BEEF

Exchanges: 3 Lean Meat, 1½ Vegetable

Serving Size: ⅔ cup
Carbohydrate: 8 gm
Protein: 25 gm
Fat: 4 gm

Calories: 172
Fiber: 2 gm
Sodium: 176 mg
Cholesterol: 64 mg

INGREDIENTS:

1 cup finely chopped onion
1 teaspoon ground ginger
1 teaspoon ground turmeric
1 teaspoon chili powder
2 cloves garlic, minced
1 pound lean boneless sirloin tip roast, trimmed and cut into ½-inch cubes

Vegetable cooking spray
1 cup water
2 teaspoons low-sodium beef-flavored bouillon granules
1 (16-ounce) can whole tomatoes, undrained and chopped

STEPS IN PREPARATION:

1. Combine first 5 ingredients in a medium bowl, stirring well. Add beef, stirring to coat. Cover and chill 2 hours.
2. Cook beef mixture in a large saucepan coated with cooking spray until all sides are browned. Stir in water, bouillon granules, and tomato. Bring to a boil; reduce heat, and simmer, covered, 1 hour.
3. Uncover and simmer an additional 30 minutes or until meat is tender and liquid is reduced.
4. Serve over cooked rice (cooked without salt or fat), if desired.

Yield: 6 servings

Note: See the Starch List on page 16 for exchange value of rice.

SLICED STEAK AU JUS

Exchanges: 2 Lean Meat

Serving Size: 2 ounces
Carbohydrate: 1 gm
Protein: 14 gm
Fat: 2 gm

Calories: 81
Fiber: 0 gm
Sodium: 140 mg
Cholesterol: 37 mg

INGREDIENTS:

1¾ pounds lean top round steak
Vegetable cooking spray
1 (3-ounce) can sliced mushrooms, drained
1 tablespoon Worcestershire sauce

1 tablespoon lemon juice
½ teaspoon salt
Dash of pepper
1 garlic clove, minced

STEPS IN PREPARATION:

1. Cut steak into ¼-inch slices; arrange slices in a shallow baking dish coated with cooking spray.
2. Sprinkle mushrooms and remaining ingredients over steak.
3. Cover and bake at 350° for 1 hour.
4. Uncover and bake an additional 15 minutes or to desired degree of doneness, basting occasionally.

Yield: 14 servings

Look for cuts of beef with "loin" or "round" in the name. They're among the leanest choices.

MARINATED STEAK

Exchanges: 2 Medium-Fat Meat

Serving Size: 2 ounces with sauce
Carbohydrate: 2 gm
Protein: 15 gm
Fat: 2 gm

Calories: 113
Fiber: 1 gm
Sodium: 261 mg
Cholesterol: 39 mg

INGREDIENTS:

1½ teaspoons Worcestershire sauce
4 (2½-ounce) lean round steaks
½ teaspoon garlic salt
½ teaspoon instant minced onion
½ teaspoon pepper
½ cup dry white wine
1 cup water
1 (3-ounce) can sliced mushrooms, drained

STEPS IN PREPARATION:

1. Spoon Worcestershire sauce over both sides of steaks. Sprinkle steaks with garlic salt, onion, and pepper. Cover and chill 1 hour.
2. Cook steaks in a nonstick skillet over medium heat until meat is browned on both sides.
3. Pour wine over steaks. Cover and reduce heat; simmer 15 minutes.
4. Remove steaks to a serving platter, and keep warm.
5. Add water and mushrooms to skillet; boil, uncovered, 10 minutes or until gravy is reduced to about ½ cup, stirring frequently. Spoon gravy over steaks, and serve.

Yield: 4 servings

Alcohol evaporates at 172°F, so when you use liqueurs, wines, and spirits in cooking, most of the alcohol evaporates, leaving only the flavor behind. However, the amount of alcohol that evaporates depends on the type of heat applied, the source of the alcohol (wine versus distilled spirits), and the cooking time.

STEAK DELUXE

Exchanges: ½ Starch, 2 Medium-Fat Meat

Serving Size: 2 ounces with sauce
Carbohydrate: 5 gm
Protein: 17 gm
Fat: 3 gm

Calories: 116
Fiber: 1 gm
Sodium: 190 mg
Cholesterol: 42 mg

INGREDIENTS:

1 pound lean round steak
2 tablespoons all-purpose flour
1 teaspoon reduced-calorie margarine
Vegetable cooking spray
1¼ cups cooked tomato
1 tablespoon granulated brown sugar substitute

2 teaspoons Worcestershire sauce
½ teaspoon celery salt
½ teaspoon vinegar
¼ teaspoon dried thyme
⅛ teaspoon garlic powder
⅛ teaspoon pepper
½ medium onion, sliced

STEPS IN PREPARATION:

1. Lightly dredge steak in flour.
2. Melt margarine in a nonstick skillet. Add steak, and cook over medium heat until steak is browned on both sides.
3. Transfer steak to a 13- x 9- x 2-inch baking dish coated with cooking spray.
4. Combine tomato and remaining ingredients; pour over steak. Cover; bake at 300° for 2½ hours. Uncover and bake an additional 15 minutes or until liquid is thickened.

Yield: 6 servings

SWISS STEAK
Exchanges: 3 Lean Meat, 2 Vegetable

Serving Size: ⅙ recipe
Carbohydrate: 7 gm
Protein: 27 gm
Fat: 5 gm

Calories: 188
Fiber: 1 gm
Sodium: 396 mg
Cholesterol: 70 mg

INGREDIENTS:

1½ pounds lean round steak, trimmed and cut into 6 pieces
1 tablespoon reduced-calorie margarine, melted
1 (16-ounce) can stewed tomatoes, undrained
1 small onion, sliced

1 stalk celery, sliced
1 medium carrot, scraped and thinly sliced
1 teaspoon Worcestershire sauce
1 tablespoon all-purpose flour
½ teaspoon salt
¼ cup water

STEPS IN PREPARATION:

1. Place each piece of steak between two sheets of heavy-duty plastic wrap, and flatten to ¼-inch thickness, using a meat mallet or rolling pin.
2. Cook meat in margarine in a large skillet over medium heat until both sides are browned. Drain and pat dry with paper towels.
3. Return meat to skillet; add stewed tomatoes and next 4 ingredients. Cover and cook over low heat 1 hour and 15 minutes or until meat is tender. Transfer meat to a serving platter, and keep warm.
4. Skim excess fat from tomato mixture. Combine flour and salt; add water, and stir until well blended. Stir into tomato mixture. Cook over medium heat 2 minutes or until thickened and bubbly, stirring frequently. Remove tomato mixture from heat; spoon over meat.

Yield: 6 servings

STIR-FRIED BEEF

Exchanges: 1 Lean Meat, 1 Vegetable

Serving Size: ½ cup
Carbohydrate: 6 gm
Protein: 11 gm
Fat: 1 gm

Calories: 81
Fiber: 1 gm
Sodium: 381 mg
Cholesterol: 24 mg

INGREDIENTS:

1 pound lean boneless top round steak, trimmed
⅔ cup water
¼ cup chopped onion
3 tablespoons reduced-sodium soy sauce
1 teaspoon beef-flavored bouillon granules
1 teaspoon Worcestershire sauce
½ teaspoon salt

⅛ teaspoon pepper
1 clove garlic, minced
2 cups cauliflower flowerets
2 medium carrots, scraped and diagonally sliced
Vegetable cooking spray
1 cup sliced fresh mushrooms
1 (6-ounce) package frozen snow pea pods, thawed
¼ cup water
1 tablespoon cornstarch

STEPS IN PREPARATION:

1. Partially freeze steak; slice diagonally across grain into ¼-inch strips. Set aside.
2. Combine ⅔ cup water and next 7 ingredients. Add steak, stirring to coat. Cover and chill 1 hour. Drain steak, reserving marinade.
3. Cook cauliflower and carrot in boiling water to cover 3 minutes; drain and set aside.
4. Coat a wok or large skillet with cooking spray; heat at medium-high (375°) 2 minutes. Add steak; stir-fry 3 minutes. Add mushrooms; stir-fry 1 minute. Add snow peas, carrot, and cauliflower; stir-fry 2 minutes or until vegetables are crisp-tender.
5. Combine reserved marinade, ¼ cup water, and cornstarch, stirring to blend. Pour over steak mixture, and stir-fry until thickened.
6. Serve over cooked rice (cooked without salt or fat), if desired.

Yield: 12 servings

Note: See the Starch List on page 16 for exchange value of rice.

BEEF STEW

Exchanges: 2 Starch, 2 Lean Meat, 1 Vegetable

Serving Size: 1 cup
Carbohydrate: 31 gm
Protein: 22 gm
Fat: 3 gm

Calories: 240
Fiber: 5 gm
Sodium: 887 mg
Cholesterol: 45 mg

INGREDIENTS:

1 pound lean beef, cubed
2 tablespoons Worcestershire sauce
½ teaspoon salt
¼ teaspoon dried oregano
⅛ teaspoon ground allspice
1 beef bouillon cube
2 cups boiling water
1 cup canned tomatoes, undrained
4 medium baking potatoes, cubed
3 medium carrots, sliced
3 small onions, quartered
1 (10-ounce) package frozen English peas

STEPS IN PREPARATION:

1. Marinate beef in Worcestershire sauce 4 hours.
2. Cook beef in a nonstick skillet over medium heat until browned on all sides. Add salt, oregano, and allspice.
3. Dissolve bouillon cube in boiling water; add to beef mixture. Add tomatoes, and cook over low heat 1½ to 2 hours or until meat is tender.
4. Add potato, carrot, and onion; cook 30 minutes.
5. Add peas; cook an additional 15 minutes or until vegetables are tender.

Yield: 6 servings

POT ROAST WITH VEGETABLES

Exchanges: 1 Starch, 3 Medium-Fat Meat

Serving Size: ⅙ recipe
Carbohydrate: 19 gm
Protein: 22 gm
Fat: 12 gm

Calories: 269
Fiber: 3 gm
Sodium: 195 mg
Cholesterol: 60 mg

INGREDIENTS:

1 pound lean boneless chuck roast, trimmed
Vegetable cooking spray
¼ cup water
¼ teaspoon salt
⅛ teaspoon pepper
2 medium onions, peeled and sliced

2 stalks celery, sliced
4 large carrots, scraped and sliced
2 medium-size red round potatoes, peeled and cubed

STEPS IN PREPARATION:

1. Cook roast over medium heat in a small Dutch oven coated with cooking spray until browned on all sides. Add water and next 4 ingredients. Cover and bake at 350° for 1 hour and 15 minutes.
2. Add carrot and potato; bake an additional hour or until meat and vegetables are tender.
3. Transfer meat and vegetables to a serving platter; cut roast into 2-ounce slices.

Yield: 6 servings

VEAL PARMIGIANA

Exchanges: 2 Lean Meat, 1 Vegetable

Serving Size: ⅙ recipe	**Calories:** 145
Carbohydrate: 6 gm	**Fiber:** 1 gm
Protein: 17 gm	**Sodium:** 555 mg
Fat: 5 gm	**Cholesterol:** 87 mg

INGREDIENTS:

1 egg, lightly beaten
½ teaspoon salt
¼ teaspoon pepper
¼ cup soft breadcrumbs
1 tablespoon grated
   Parmesan cheese

1 pound thin veal cutlets, cut
   into 6 pieces
Vegetable cooking spray
1 (8-ounce) can tomato sauce
2 (1-ounce) slices part-skim
   mozzarella cheese

STEPS IN PREPARATION:

1. Combine egg, salt, and pepper; beat with a wire whisk until blended. Combine breadcrumbs and Parmesan cheese in a shallow dish, stirring well. Dip veal into egg mixture, and dredge in breadcrumb mixture.
2. Cook veal over medium heat in a large skillet coated with cooking spray until lightly browned on both sides.
3. Transfer veal to a shallow baking dish coated with cooking spray. Pour tomato sauce over veal. Bake at 350° for 15 minutes. Top with cheese slices, and bake an additional 5 minutes. Serve immediately.

Yield: 6 servings

Because veal comes from young animals, it does not have the marbling (fat) that is found in other good cuts of meat. Most cuts of veal are considered lean, with the leg, shoulder, loin, and sirloin being the leanest.

VEAL SCALLOPINI

Exchanges: 2 Medium-Fat Meat, 1 Vegetable

Serving Size: ½ cup
Carbohydrate: 5 gm
Protein: 15 gm
Fat: 5 gm

Calories: 120
Fiber: 1 gm
Sodium: 523 mg
Cholesterol: 54 mg

INGREDIENTS:

½ cup chopped onion
¼ cup chopped green pepper
1 tablespoon reduced-calorie margarine, melted
1 pound veal cutlets, sliced into thin strips
1 cup canned tomato sauce

1 cup water
¼ teaspoon salt
¼ teaspoon dried thyme
⅛ teaspoon pepper
½ cup (2 ounces) shredded low-fat process American cheese

STEPS IN PREPARATION:

1. Sauté onion and green pepper in margarine in a nonstick skillet until tender; remove from skillet, and set aside.
2. Place veal in skillet, and cook over medium heat until browned on both sides.
3. Add tomato sauce and next 4 ingredients. Return onion and green pepper to skillet. Cover; simmer 15 minutes.
4. Remove from heat, and sprinkle with cheese.
5. Serve over spaghetti noodles (cooked without salt or fat), if desired.

Yield: 6 servings

Note: See the Starch List on page 16 for exchange value of noodles.

PORK CHOPS WITH APPLES

Exchanges: 3 Lean Meat, 1 Fruit

Serving Size: 1 chop with apple
Carbohydrate: 17 gm
Protein: 26 gm
Fat: 9 gm

Calories: 253
Fiber: 2 gm
Sodium: 363 mg
Cholesterol: 72 mg

INGREDIENTS:

4 (4-ounce) lean boneless
  center-cut pork chops
1 medium onion, chopped
Vegetable cooking spray
1¼ cups water
1 teaspoon chicken-flavored
  bouillon granules

¼ teaspoon pepper
3 medium cooking apples,
  peeled and sliced
½ teaspoon ground cinnamon

STEPS IN PREPARATION:

1. Cook pork chops and onion in a large skillet coated with cooking spray over medium heat until pork is lightly browned.
2. Combine water, bouillon granules, and pepper, stirring until granules dissolve; add to skillet.
3. Cover and bring to a boil. Reduce heat, and simmer 20 minutes. Skim off fat.
4. Add apple slices and cinnamon to skillet. Cover and simmer 15 minutes or until pork is tender.
Yield: 4 servings

PORK CHOP DINNER

Exchanges: 2 Starch, 3 Medium-Fat Meat

Serving Size: 1 chop with rice
Carbohydrate: 29 gm
Protein: 24 gm
Fat: 11 gm

Calories: 319
Fiber: 2 gm
Sodium: 1047 mg
Cholesterol: 69 mg

INGREDIENTS:

4 (6-ounce) lean center-cut
  pork chops (½ inch thick)
¼ cup chopped onion
¼ cup chopped green pepper
1½ cups canned tomatoes
½ cup long-grain rice,
  uncooked

1 teaspoon salt
¼ teaspoon dry mustard
⅛ teaspoon ground allspice
⅛ teaspoon pepper

STEPS IN PREPARATION:

1. Cook pork chops in a nonstick skillet over medium heat until lightly browned. Drain and pat dry with paper towels. Set chops aside.
2. Sauté onion and green pepper in skillet until tender.
3. Combine tomatoes and remaining ingredients; add to skillet.
4. Place pork chops on top of mixture in skillet. Cover; simmer 30 minutes or until rice is tender.

Yield: 4 servings

CREOLE PORK CHOPS

Exchanges: 2 Medium-Fat Meat, 2 Vegetable

Serving Size: 1 chop with sauce
Carbohydrate: 9 gm
Protein: 20 gm
Fat: 10 gm

Calories: 201
Fiber: 2 gm
Sodium: 555 mg
Cholesterol: 60 mg

INGREDIENTS:

4 (3-ounce) lean boneless
   pork chops
1 (16-ounce) can crushed
   tomatoes
⅓ cup chopped onion
¼ cup chopped green pepper

¼ cup chopped celery
½ teaspoon salt
½ teaspoon hot sauce
¼ teaspoon dried oregano
1 bay leaf

STEPS IN PREPARATION:

1. Cook chops in a nonstick skillet over medium heat until lightly browned. Drain and pat dry with paper towels.
2. Return chops to skillet. Add tomatoes and remaining ingredients; cover and simmer 1 hour or until chops are tender.
3. To serve, remove and discard bay leaf. Spoon sauce evenly over chops.

Yield: 4 servings

SWEET-AND-SOUR PORK

Exchanges: 1 Lean Meat, 1 Vegetable

Serving Size: ½ cup
Carbohydrate: 8 gm
Protein: 11 gm
Fat: 2 gm

Calories: 97
Fiber: trace
Sodium: 458 mg
Cholesterol: 44 mg

INGREDIENTS:

1½ cups fat-free chicken broth, divided
1 tablespoon cornstarch
1 tablespoon all-purpose flour
½ teaspoon salt
1 egg
1 pound lean boneless pork, trimmed and cubed
Vegetable cooking spray
½ cup chopped carrot

1 medium-size green pepper, chopped
1 clove garlic, minced
⅓ cup red wine vinegar
2 tablespoons reduced-sodium soy sauce
1 tablespoon cornstarch
¼ cup water
Sugar substitute to equal ¾ cup sugar*

STEPS IN PREPARATION:

1. Combine ¼ cup broth, 1 tablespoon cornstarch, and next 3 ingredients; beat with a wire whisk. Dip pork cubes into mixture.
2. Coat a skillet with cooking spray; place over medium heat until hot. Add pork; cook 5 minutes. Remove pork; drain.
3. Wipe skillet with a paper towel; coat skillet with cooking spray. Add carrot, pepper, and garlic; sauté until tender. Stir in remaining 1¼ cups broth, vinegar, and soy sauce.
4. Dissolve 1 tablespoon cornstarch in water. Stir into vegetable mixture, and bring to a boil. Reduce heat, and simmer, stirring constantly, 1 to 2 minutes or until vegetable mixture is thickened. Stir in pork and sugar substitute. Cover and simmer until pork is tender.
5. Serve over cooked rice (cooked without salt or fat), if desired.

Yield: 10 servings

Note: See the Starch List on page 16 for exchange value of rice.

*See the sugar substitution chart on page 354.

HAM AND CORN CASSEROLE

Exchanges: 2 Starch, 2 Medium-Fat Meat

Serving Size: ¾ cup	**Calories:** 256
Carbohydrate: 29 gm	**Fiber:** 2 gm
Protein: 17 gm	**Sodium:** 1203 mg
Fat: 9 gm	**Cholesterol:** 30 mg

INGREDIENTS:

3 tablespoons all-purpose flour
1½ cups skim milk, divided
3 tablespoons reduced-calorie margarine
2 cups cubed lean cooked ham
¼ cup chopped onion
¼ cup chopped green pepper
½ teaspoon dry mustard
¼ teaspoon salt
¼ teaspoon Worcestershire sauce
⅛ teaspoon pepper
1 (20-ounce) can whole kernel corn, drained
Vegetable cooking spray
1 cup soft breadcrumbs
1 cup (4 ounces) shredded low-fat process American cheese

STEPS IN PREPARATION:

1. Combine flour and ½ cup milk; stir until smooth. Combine flour mixture, remaining 1 cup milk, and margarine in a small saucepan; stir well. Cook over medium heat, stirring constantly, until mixture is thickened and bubbly.
2. Stir in ham and next 7 ingredients.
3. Spoon mixture into a 1½-quart casserole coated with cooking spray. Top with breadcrumbs and cheese. Bake at 375° for 25 minutes or until bubbly.

Yield: 8 servings

BAKED HAM WITH PINEAPPLE

Exchanges: 2 Lean Meat, ½ Fruit

Serving Size: ¹/₁₂ recipe	**Calories:** 122
Carbohydrate: 4 gm	**Fiber:** trace
Protein: 16 gm	**Sodium:** 910 mg
Fat: 4 gm	**Cholesterol:** 40 mg

INGREDIENTS:

1 (2-pound) fully cooked boneless smoked ham
20 whole cloves
4 slices canned pineapple in juice, drained
½ cup sugar-free ginger ale
1 teaspoon ground cinnamon

STEPS IN PREPARATION:

1. Remove and discard casing from ham. Score top of ham in a diamond design, and stud with cloves.
2. Place ham in a shallow baking dish, and arrange pineapple slices over ham. Pour ginger ale over ham, and sprinkle pineapple slices evenly with cinnamon. Bake at 325° for 25 to 30 minutes or until thoroughly heated.
3. To serve, cut into 12 slices.

Yield: 12 servings

Reduced-fat cooked hams are now available. Look for them in the meat section of your local supermarket.

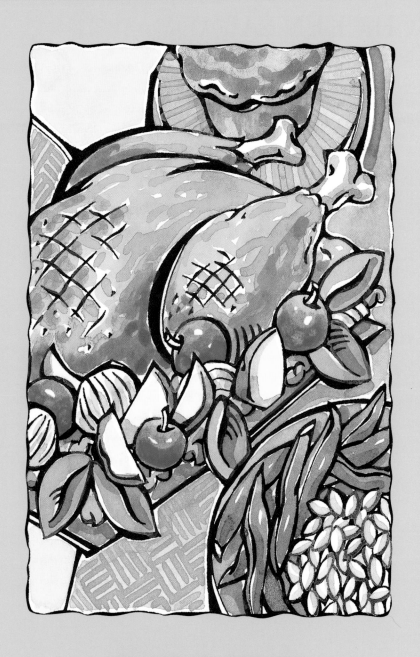

POULTRY

CHICKEN SALAD

Exchanges: 2 Lean Meat, 2 Vegetable

Serving Size: ¾ cup	**Calories:** 118
Carbohydrate: 10 gm	**Fiber:** 1 gm
Protein: 15 gm	**Sodium:** 796 mg
Fat: 2 gm	**Cholesterol:** 36 mg

INGREDIENTS:

2 cups diced cooked chicken
   (skinned before cooking
   and cooked without salt)
1 cup finely chopped celery
¾ cup reduced-calorie
   mayonnaise
⅔ cup chopped onion

1 tablespoon chopped
   pimiento
1 teaspoon salt
1 teaspoon Worcestershire
   sauce
¼ teaspoon pepper
Lettuce leaves (optional)

STEPS IN PREPARATION:

1. Combine first 8 ingredients; stir well. Cover and chill.
2. Serve on lettuce leaves, if desired.

Yield: 6 servings

For every chicken breast half, you can count on
getting about ½ cup of chopped or diced chicken.

CHICKEN CASSEROLE

Exchanges: 1 Lean Meat, 1 Vegetable

Serving Size: ½ cup
Carbohydrate: 6 gm
Protein: 14 gm
Fat: 4 gm

Calories: 120
Fiber: trace
Sodium: 367 mg
Cholesterol: 32 mg

INGREDIENTS:

4 (3-ounce) skinned chicken breast halves
4 cups water
Vegetable cooking spray
¼ teaspoon salt
¼ teaspoon pepper
½ cup skim milk

½ (8-ounce) carton plain low-fat yogurt
½ (10½-ounce) can cream of chicken soup, undiluted
5 unsalted crackers, crushed
1 teaspoon reduced-calorie margarine, melted

STEPS IN PREPARATION:

1. Combine chicken breast halves and water in a medium saucepan; cover and bring to a boil. Reduce heat, and simmer 15 to 20 minutes or until chicken is done; drain well. Remove chicken from bone; coarsely chop chicken.
2. Place chopped chicken in a 1-quart casserole coated with cooking spray, and sprinkle with salt and pepper.
3. Combine milk, yogurt, and soup in a medium bowl, stirring until well blended; spoon mixture evenly over chicken.
4. Combine crushed crackers and melted margarine, stirring well. Sprinkle cracker mixture evenly over top of casserole. Bake at 350° for 20 minutes or until thoroughly heated.

Yield: 6 servings

CHICKEN-CAULIFLOWER CASSEROLE

Exchanges: 1 Lean Meat, 1½ Vegetable

Serving Size: ¾ cup	**Calories:** 106
Carbohydrate: 8 gm	**Fiber:** 1 gm
Protein: 11 gm	**Sodium:** 296 mg
Fat: 3 gm	**Cholesterol:** 22 mg

INGREDIENTS:

1 (10-ounce) package frozen chopped cauliflower
½ cup coarsely chopped onion
½ cup water
1 cup skim milk
1 tablespoon cornstarch
1 teaspoon low-sodium chicken-flavored bouillon granules
½ teaspoon salt
¼ cup (1 ounce) shredded low-fat process American cheese
1 cup chopped cooked chicken (skinned before cooking and cooked without salt)
1 (4-ounce) jar diced pimiento, drained
Vegetable cooking spray

STEPS IN PREPARATION:

1. Combine cauliflower, onion, and water in a medium saucepan; cover and bring to a boil. Reduce heat, and simmer 5 minutes or until vegetables are tender. Drain well, and set aside.
2. Add milk, cornstarch, bouillon granules, and salt to saucepan, stirring with a wire whisk. Bring to a boil; reduce heat, and simmer, stirring constantly, until thickened and bubbly.
3. Add cheese; stir with wire whisk until cheese melts. Remove from heat.
4. Add cauliflower mixture, chicken, and pimiento to cheese sauce. Spoon mixture into a 1½-quart casserole coated with cooking spray. Bake at 325° for 20 minutes or until thoroughly heated.

Yield: 6 servings

CHICKEN AND RICE CASSEROLE

Exchanges: 1 Starch, 2 Medium-Fat Meat

Serving Size: ½ cup
Carbohydrate: 21 gm
Protein: 15 gm
Fat: 7 gm

Calories: 210
Fiber: 1 gm
Sodium: 839 mg
Cholesterol: 90 mg

INGREDIENTS:

1½ cups diced cooked chicken (skinned before cooking and cooked without salt)
1 cup cooked long-grain rice (cooked without salt or fat)
½ cup chopped celery
¼ cup nonfat mayonnaise
1 tablespoon lemon juice
2 hard-cooked eggs, chopped
1 (10¾-ounce) can cream of mushroom soup, undiluted
1 small onion, chopped
Vegetable cooking spray
¼ cup soft breadcrumbs
1 tablespoon dry butter substitute

STEPS IN PREPARATION:

1. Combine first 8 ingredients; stir well. Spoon mixture into a shallow 2-quart casserole coated with cooking spray.
2. Combine bread crumbs and butter substitute; sprinkle over top of casserole. Bake at 350°, uncovered, for 40 to 45 minutes or until bubbly.

Yield: 6 servings

CHICKEN TORTILLA CASSEROLE

Exchanges: 1 Starch, 2 Lean Meat

Serving Size: 1/6 recipe	**Calories:** 180
Carbohydrate: 16 gm	**Fiber:** 2 gm
Protein: 15 gm	**Sodium:** 796 mg
Fat: 7 gm	**Cholesterol:** 32 mg

INGREDIENTS:

2 (4-ounce) skinned, boned chicken breast halves
4 cups water
½ cup skim milk
½ cup chunky salsa
½ small onion, grated
½ (10½-ounce) can cream of chicken soup, undiluted
6 (6-inch) corn tortillas, cut into wedges
1 cup (4 ounces) shredded low-fat process American cheese
Vegetable cooking spray
1½ large canned green chiles, seeded and diced

STEPS IN PREPARATION:

1. Combine chicken and water in a small saucepan; cover and bring to a boil. Reduce heat, and simmer 20 minutes or until chicken is done; drain well. Chop chicken, and set aside.
2. Combine milk, salsa, onion, and soup, stirring to blend. Layer half each of tortillas, chicken, soup mixture, and cheese in a 1½-quart casserole coated with cooking spray. Sprinkle with chiles.
3. Repeat layers with remaining tortillas, chicken, soup mixture, and cheese. Cover and chill overnight.
4. Bake at 300° for 1 hour or until thoroughly heated. Divide into 6 equal portions, and serve warm.

Yield: 6 servings

CHICKEN AND VEGETABLE CASSEROLE

Exchanges: ½ Starch, 2 Medium-Fat Meat, 1 Vegetable

Serving Size: 1 cup
Carbohydrate: 7 gm
Protein: 24 gm
Fat: 3 gm

Calories: 168
Fiber: 0 gm
Sodium: 129 mg
Cholesterol: 28 mg

INGREDIENTS:

1 (10¾-ounce) can cream of mushroom soup, undiluted
¼ cup skim milk
1 teaspoon Worcestershire sauce
1 cup diced cooked chicken (skinned before cooking and cooked without salt)

1 cup cooked sliced okra
¼ cup chopped celery
¼ cup chopped green pepper
Vegetable cooking spray

STEPS IN PREPARATION:

1. Combine first 3 ingredients in a medium bowl.
2. Add chicken, okra, celery, and green pepper.
3. Spoon mixture into a 1-quart casserole coated with cooking spray. Bake at 350° for 20 minutes or until thoroughly heated.

Yield: 4 servings

BOMBAY CHICKEN

Exchanges: ½ Starch, 2 Lean Meat

Serving Size: ½ cup
Carbohydrate: 11 gm
Protein: 12 gm
Fat: 6 gm

Calories: 138
Fiber: 2 gm
Sodium: 300 mg
Cholesterol: 22 mg

INGREDIENTS:

1 teaspoon reduced-calorie margarine
¼ cup chopped almonds
2 teaspoons curry powder, divided
1 cup diced apple
½ cup chopped onion
½ cup sliced fresh mushrooms
1 tablespoon all-purpose flour

1 teaspoon chicken-flavored bouillon granules
1 cup boiling water
½ cup skim milk
1 tablespoon lemon juice
1 cup chopped cooked chicken (skinned before cooking and cooked without salt)

STEPS IN PREPARATION:

1. Melt margarine in a large skillet over medium heat; add almonds. Cook 10 minutes or until almonds are golden, stirring frequently. Sprinkle almonds with 1 teaspoon curry powder; toss lightly to coat. Drain almonds on paper towels.
2. Add apple, onion, and mushrooms to skillet; sauté 5 minutes. Stir in remaining 1 teaspoon curry powder and flour. Cook over low heat 2 minutes, stirring frequently.
3. Dissolve bouillon granules in boiling water; add to skillet. Stir in milk and lemon juice. Cook over low heat, stirring constantly, 5 minutes or until thickened.
4. Add chicken; cook over low heat, stirring constantly, until thoroughly heated.

Yield: 5 servings

CURRIED CHICKEN

Exchanges: 2 Lean Meat, 1 Vegetable

Serving Size: ½ cup
Carbohydrate: 9 gm
Protein: 13 gm
Fat: 3 gm

Calories: 118
Fiber: 1 gm
Sodium: 209 mg
Cholesterol: 28 mg

INGREDIENTS:

1 large apple, chopped
¼ cup sliced green onions
1 tablespoon curry powder
1 tablespoon water
1 cup skim milk
2 tablespoons minced fresh parsley

½ (10¾-ounce) can cream of mushroom soup, undiluted
2 cups chopped cooked chicken (skinned before cooking and cooked without salt)
½ cup plain low-fat yogurt

STEPS IN PREPARATION:

1. Combine first 4 ingredients in a medium saucepan; cover and cook over medium heat until onions are tender.
2. Add milk, parsley, and soup, stirring well. Add chicken; cook 10 minutes.
3. Remove from heat, and stir in yogurt.
4. Serve over cooked rice (cooked without salt or fat), if desired.

Yield: 8 servings

Note: See the Starch List on page 16 for exchange value of rice.

CHICKEN CHOW MEIN

Exchanges: 1 Lean Meat, 1 Vegetable

Serving Size: ½ cup
Carbohydrate: 5 gm
Protein: 7 gm
Fat: 1 gm

Calories: 58
Fiber: 1 gm
Sodium: 340 mg
Cholesterol: 31 mg

INGREDIENTS:

Vegetable cooking spray
1½ cups chopped onion
1 cup sliced celery
½ cup chopped green pepper
2 cups chopped cooked chicken
(skinned before cooking and
cooked without salt)
1 (14-ounce) can Chinese-style
vegetables, drained

1 (4-ounce) can sliced
mushrooms, drained
¼ teaspoon ground cumin
1 tablespoon low-sodium
chicken-flavored bouillon
granules
3 cups water, divided
1 tablespoon cornstarch

STEPS IN PREPARATION:

1. Coat a large skillet with cooking spray; place over medium heat until hot. Add onion, celery, and green pepper; sauté 3 minutes or until vegetables are tender.
2. Stir in chicken and next 3 ingredients; cook over medium heat 1 minute.
3. Add bouillon granules and 2¾ cups water to chicken mixture. Cook over medium heat, stirring constantly, until granules dissolve.
4. Combine cornstarch and remaining ¼ cup water, stirring until smooth. Add cornstarch mixture to chicken mixture; cook over medium heat, stirring constantly, until thickened and bubbly.
5. Serve over cooked rice (cooked without salt or fat), if desired.

Yield: 14 servings

Note: See the Starch List on page 16 for exchange value of rice.

CHICKEN CACCIATORE

Exchanges: 1 Lean Meat, 2 Vegetable

Serving Size: 1 cup	**Calories:** 119
Carbohydrate: 12 gm	**Fiber:** 4 gm
Protein: 13 gm	**Sodium:** 412 mg
Fat: 3 gm	**Cholesterol:** 25 mg

INGREDIENTS:

- 1 tablespoon reduced-calorie margarine
- ½ pound skinned, boned chicken breast halves
- ½ cup chopped onion
- ½ cup chopped celery
- 1 clove garlic, minced
- 1 cup sliced fresh mushrooms
- ½ cup chopped fresh parsley
- ¼ cup chopped green pepper
- 1 teaspoon dried basil
- 1 teaspoon dried oregano
- ¼ teaspoon salt
- ¼ teaspoon black pepper
- ⅛ teaspoon ground red pepper
- 1 (28-ounce) can whole tomatoes, undrained and chopped

STEPS IN PREPARATION:

1. Melt margarine over low heat in a large skillet; add chicken, and cook until lightly browned. Chop chicken, and set aside.
2. Add onion, celery, and garlic to margarine in skillet; sauté until vegetables are tender.
3. Return chicken to skillet; add mushrooms and remaining ingredients. Cover and simmer 20 minutes.
4. Serve over cooked rice or noodles (cooked without salt or fat), if desired.

Yield: 5 servings

Note: See the Starch List on page 16 for exchange values of rice and noodles.

CHICKEN SPAGHETTI

Exchanges: 1 Starch, 2½ Lean Meat

Serving Size: 1 cup
Carbohydrate: 14 gm
Protein: 20 gm
Fat: 4 gm

Calories: 176
Fiber: trace
Sodium: 363 mg
Cholesterol: 44 mg

INGREDIENTS:

1½ pounds skinned, boned
   chicken breast halves
8 cups water
4 ounces spaghetti, uncooked
½ cup skim milk
½ teaspoon salt

¼ teaspoon pepper
½ (10¾-ounce) can cream of
   mushroom soup, undiluted
1 (2-ounce) jar sliced
   mushrooms, drained
Vegetable cooking spray

STEPS IN PREPARATION:

1. Combine chicken and water in a large skillet; cover and bring to a
   boil. Reduce heat, and simmer 15 to 20 minutes or until done;
   drain well. Chop chicken, and set aside.
2. Cook spaghetti according to package directions, omitting salt and
   fat; drain, and set aside.
3. Combine milk and next 3 ingredients, stirring to blend.
4. Layer spaghetti, chicken, soup mixture, and mushrooms in a
   13- x 9- x 2-inch baking dish coated with cooking spray. Bake at
   325° for 30 to 45 minutes or until thoroughly heated.

Yield: 8 servings

BAKED CHICKEN

Exchanges: 2 Lean Meat, 1½ Vegetable

Serving Size: 1 breast half	**Calories:** 128
Carbohydrate: 8 gm	**Fiber:** 2 gm
Protein: 18 gm	**Sodium:** 180 mg
Fat: 2 gm	**Cholesterol:** 43 mg

INGREDIENTS:

4 (3-ounce) skinned, boned chicken breast halves
Vegetable cooking spray
1 (12-ounce) can whole tomatoes, undrained and chopped
½ cup chopped green pepper
½ cup chopped onion
½ teaspoon garlic powder
¼ teaspoon dried basil
¼ teaspoon dried oregano
¼ teaspoon pepper

STEPS IN PREPARATION:

1. Arrange chicken breast halves in an 11- x 7- x 2-inch baking dish coated with cooking spray.
2. Combine tomato and remaining ingredients, stirring well; spoon over chicken in dish.
3. Cover and bake at 400° for 1 hour or until chicken is done.

Yield: 4 servings

A 3-ounce portion of skinned cooked dark meat chicken has twice the fat of a 3-ounce portion of skinned cooked white meat.

BAKED CHICKEN WITH RICE

Exchanges: 2 Starch, 2 Medium-Fat Meat

Serving Size: 1 breast half
Carbohydrate: 34 gm
Protein: 30 gm
Fat: 8 gm

Calories: 336
Fiber: 1 gm
Sodium: 1057 mg
Cholesterol: 67 mg

INGREDIENTS:

1 cup long-grain rice,
   uncooked
Vegetable cooking spray
1 (1-ounce) package onion
   soup mix, divided
6 (3-ounce) skinned, boned
   chicken breast halves

1 (10¾-ounce) can cream of
   mushroom soup, undiluted
1½ cups water
⅛ teaspoon pepper

STEPS IN PREPARATION:

1. Spread rice evenly in bottom of a 9-inch square baking dish coated with cooking spray. Sprinkle with one-fourth of onion soup mix.
2. Place chicken on top of rice. Add remaining onion soup mix.
3. Combine mushroom soup, water, and pepper. Pour mushroom soup mixture over chicken. Cover and bake at 325° for 2 hours or until chicken is done.

Yield: 6 servings

CREOLE CHICKEN

Exchanges: 2 Lean Meat, 2 Vegetable

Serving Size: 1 breast half
Carbohydrate: 9 gm
Protein: 13 gm
Fat: 2 gm

Calories: 103
Fiber: 2 gm
Sodium: 491 mg
Cholesterol: 29 mg

INGREDIENTS:

4 (3-ounce) skinned, boned
  chicken breast halves
Vegetable cooking spray
½ cup chopped celery
⅓ cup sliced onion
½ teaspoon salt

½ teaspoon dried thyme
⅛ teaspoon pepper
1 medium-size green pepper,
  cut into strips
1 (16-ounce) can crushed
  tomatoes

STEPS IN PREPARATION:

1. Place chicken breasts on rack of a broiler pan coated with cooking spray. Broil 5 inches from heat 10 minutes or until lightly browned, turning once.
2. Combine celery and remaining ingredients in a large nonstick skillet. Bring mixture to a boil; cover and cook over medium heat 10 minutes.
3. Add chicken; cover and reduce heat. Simmer 30 minutes or until chicken is tender.

Yield: 4 servings

CHICKEN DIJON

Exchanges: ½ Starch, 2 Lean Meat

Serving Size: 1 breast half
Carbohydrate: 6 gm
Protein: 19 gm
Fat: 3 gm

Calories: 133
Fiber: trace
Sodium: 194 mg
Cholesterol: 44 mg

INGREDIENTS:

¼ cup Dijon mustard
½ (8-ounce) carton plain
  nonfat yogurt
8 (3-ounce) skinned chicken
  breast halves

½ cup soft breadcrumbs
Vegetable cooking spray

STEPS IN PREPARATION:

1. Combine mustard and yogurt, stirring until well blended. Brush chicken breast halves evenly with yogurt mixture, and dredge in breadcrumbs.
2. Arrange chicken in a 13- x 9- x 2-inch baking dish coated with cooking spray. Cover and bake at 400° for 30 minutes.
3. Increase temperature to 450°. Bake, uncovered, for 15 minutes or until lightly browned.

Yield: 8 servings

HERBED CHICKEN

Exchanges: 2 Lean Meat

Serving Size: 1 breast half
Carbohydrate: trace
Protein: 12 gm
Fat: 2 gm

Calories: 64
Fiber: 0 gm
Sodium: 492 mg
Cholesterol: 29 mg

INGREDIENTS:

6 (4-ounce) skinned chicken
  breast halves
Vegetable cooking spray
2 teaspoons dried rosemary

½ teaspoon salt
¼ teaspoon pepper
2 chicken bouillon cubes
1 cup water

STEPS IN PREPARATION:

1. Place chicken in a shallow baking dish coated with cooking spray. Sprinkle with rosemary, salt, and pepper.
2. Crumble bouillon cubes between pieces of chicken.
3. Add water to baking dish.
4. Cover and bake at 350° for 1 hour or until chicken is done. Uncover and bake an additional 5 minutes or until chicken is lightly browned.

Yield: 6 servings

Cooking with herbs? Use finely chopped fresh herbs whenever possible for the best flavor. When substituting, use three times as much fresh herbs as dried herbs.

GRILLED MARINATED CHICKEN

Exchanges: 2 Lean Meat

Serving Size: 1 breast half
Carbohydrate: 4 gm
Protein: 14 gm
Fat: 3 gm

Calories: 108
Fiber: trace
Sodium: 240 mg
Cholesterol: 36 mg

INGREDIENTS:

6 (3-ounce) skinned chicken
   breast halves
Sugar substitute to equal ¼
   cup plus 2 tablespoons
   sugar*
3 tablespoons lemon juice

3 tablespoons vinegar
2 tablespoons reduced-calorie
   mayonnaise
½ teaspoon salt
½ teaspoon pepper
Vegetable cooking spray

STEPS IN PREPARATION:

1. Place chicken in a shallow dish.
2. Combine sugar substitute and next 5 ingredients, stirring well. Pour over chicken. Cover and marinate in refrigerator at least 1 hour.
3. Remove chicken from marinade, reserving marinade. Coat grill rack with cooking spray; place on grill over hot coals (400° to 500°). Place chicken on rack; grill, uncovered, for 45 minutes or until done. Turn and baste every 10 minutes with reserved marinade.

Yield: 6 servings

*See the sugar substitution chart on page 354.

OVEN-FRIED CHICKEN

Exchanges: ½ Starch, 3 Lean Meat

Serving Size: 1 breast half	**Calories:** 155
Carbohydrate: 7 gm	**Fiber:** 0 gm
Protein: 24 gm	**Sodium:** 129 mg
Fat: 3 gm	**Cholesterol:** 58 mg

INGREDIENTS:

1 cup crushed corn flakes
    cereal
¼ teaspoon paprika
¼ teaspoon onion powder
¼ teaspoon garlic powder

¼ teaspoon curry powder
4 (4-ounce) skinned chicken
    breast halves
4 teaspoons skim milk
Vegetable cooking spray

STEPS IN PREPARATION:

1. Combine first 5 ingredients in a shallow dish.
2. Dip chicken in milk, and dredge in cereal mixture.
3. Place chicken in a small baking dish coated with cooking spray.
   Bake at 350° for 20 to 30 minutes or until lightly browned.

Yield: 4 servings

Chicken with a crisp oven-fried coating and low-fat gravy offers a satisfying yet healthier alternative to pan- or deep-fried chicken.

SOY CHICKEN

Exchanges: ½ Starch, 3 Lean Meat

Serving Size: 1 breast half	**Calories:** 162
Carbohydrate: 4 gm	**Fiber:** 0 gm
Protein: 27 gm	**Sodium:** 1105 mg
Fat: 3 gm	**Cholesterol:** 66 mg

INGREDIENTS:

6 (4-ounce) skinned chicken
  breast halves
Dash of onion powder
Dash of garlic powder

⅓ cup soy sauce
⅓ cup Worcestershire sauce
⅓ cup vinegar
⅓ cup water

STEPS IN PREPARATION:

1. Sprinkle both sides of chicken with onion and garlic powders. Place chicken in a shallow baking dish.
2. Combine soy sauce and remaining ingredients. Pour soy sauce mixture over chicken.
3. Cover and chill at least 3 hours.
4. Bake, uncovered, at 350° for 1 hour or until chicken is tender.

Yield: 6 servings

If you need to reduce sodium, use low-sodium soy sauce and low-sodium Worcestershire sauce instead of the regular products.

SQUASH MIX WITH CHICKEN

Exchanges: 1 Lean Meat, 2 Vegetable

Serving Size: 1 cup	**Calories:** 78
Carbohydrate: 10 gm	**Fiber:** 3 gm
Protein: 7 gm	**Sodium:** 311 mg
Fat: 1 gm	**Cholesterol:** 14 mg

INGREDIENTS:

½ cup chopped onion
½ cup sliced celery
1 teaspoon reduced-calorie
  margarine, melted
2½ cups sliced yellow squash
1 cup sliced zucchini
½ cup chopped cooked chicken
  (skinned before cooking and
  cooked without salt)

2 tablespoons water
½ teaspoon salt
½ teaspoon dried chervil
⅛ teaspoon ground red
  pepper
⅛ teaspoon black pepper

STEPS IN PREPARATION:

1. Sauté onion and celery in margarine in a large skillet until tender. Stir in squash and remaining ingredients. Cover and bring to a boil.
2. Reduce heat, and simmer 8 to 10 minutes or until vegetables are tender, stirring frequently.
3. Transfer mixture to a serving dish, and serve warm.

Yield: 4 servings

CHICKEN TOSTADA WITH SALSA

Exchanges: 1 Starch, 2 Lean Meat

Serving Size: 1 tortilla half	**Calories:** 172
Carbohydrate: 16 gm	**Fiber:** 1 gm
Protein: 14 gm	**Sodium:** 336 mg
Fat: 6 gm	**Cholesterol:** 31 mg

INGREDIENTS:

1 tablespoon vegetable oil
4 (8-inch) flour tortillas
3 cups shredded lettuce
2 medium tomatoes
¼ cup chopped green onions
2 cups shredded cooked chicken (skinned before cooking and cooked without salt)

¼ cup (1 ounce) shredded low-fat process American cheese
1 cup Salsa (see page 296)

STEPS IN PREPARATION:

1. Place oil in a large skillet, and place skillet over medium heat until oil is hot.
2. Add tortillas, one at a time, and cook 1 minute on each side or until thoroughly heated. Cut each tortilla in half.
3. Spoon lettuce evenly onto tortilla halves. Cut each tomato into 8 wedges, and arrange on lettuce. Sprinkle evenly with onions, and top evenly with shredded chicken and cheese. Spoon 2 tablespoons Salsa over each tortilla half.

Yield: 8 servings

CHICKEN CORDON BLEU

Exchanges: 3 Lean Meat, 1 Vegetable

Serving Size: 1 chicken roll
Carbohydrate: 7 gm
Protein: 21 gm
Fat: 8 gm

Calories: 192
Fiber: trace
Sodium: 398 mg
Cholesterol: 98 mg

INGREDIENTS:

4 (3-ounce) skinned, boned chicken breast halves
2 (1-ounce) slices lean cooked ham, cut in half
2 (1-ounce) slices low-fat process Swiss cheese, cut in half

1 egg, lightly beaten
2 tablespoons all-purpose flour
Vegetable cooking spray
⅓ cup chopped onion
¼ (10½-ounce) can cream of chicken soup, undiluted

STEPS IN PREPARATION:

1. Place chicken between 2 sheets of heavy-duty plastic wrap, and flatten to ¼-inch thickness using a meat mallet or rolling pin.
2. Place one slice each of ham and cheese in center of each chicken breast half. Roll up lengthwise, and secure with wooden picks.
3. Dip each chicken roll in egg, and dredge in flour. Place chicken rolls, seam side down, in a shallow baking dish coated with cooking spray. Bake at 350° for 20 minutes.
4. Combine onion and soup, stirring well. Spoon over chicken, and bake at 350° for 15 minutes or until chicken is done.

Yield: 4 servings

CHICKEN DIVAN

Exchanges: 2 Lean Meat, 1 Vegetable

Serving Size: 1 cup	**Calories:** 113
Carbohydrate: 4 gm	**Fiber:** 1 gm
Protein: 17 gm	**Sodium:** 224 mg
Fat: 3 gm	**Cholesterol:** 39 mg

INGREDIENTS:

8 (3-ounce) skinned, boned
  chicken breast halves
8 cups water
1 (10-ounce) package frozen
  chopped broccoli, thawed
Vegetable cooking spray
¼ (10¾-ounce) can cream of
  chicken soup, undiluted

¼ (10¾-ounce) can cream of
  potato soup, undiluted
½ cup skim milk
1½ teaspoons lemon juice
2 tablespoons grated
  Parmesan cheese

STEPS IN PREPARATION:

1. Combine chicken and water in a large saucepan; cover and bring
   to a boil. Reduce heat, and simmer 20 minutes or until chicken is
   done; drain well. Chop chicken.
2. Place broccoli in a 2-quart baking dish coated with cooking spray;
   top with chicken.
3. Combine soups, milk, and lemon juice, stirring to blend; pour
   over chicken and broccoli. Sprinkle with cheese. Bake at 350° for
   25 minutes or until thoroughly heated.

Yield: 8 servings

CHICKEN AND DUMPLINGS

Exchanges: 1 Starch, 2 Medium-Fat Meat

Serving Size: ¾ cup
Carbohydrate: 18 gm
Protein: 14 gm
Fat: 9 gm

Calories: 213
Fiber: 1 gm
Sodium: 371 mg
Cholesterol: 33 mg

INGREDIENTS:

1 (3-pound) broiler-fryer, skinned
1½ cups water
¼ cup chopped celery
¼ cup chopped onion
¼ teaspoon salt

1 cup all-purpose flour
1 teaspoon baking powder
½ teaspoon salt
3 tablespoons vegetable shortening
¼ cup skim milk

STEPS IN PREPARATION:

1. Disjoint chicken; place in a large Dutch oven. Add water and next 3 ingredients; simmer 1 hour or until chicken is tender.
2. Combine flour, baking powder, and salt. Cut in shortening with a pastry blender. Add milk to make a stiff dough. Roll dough out to ⅛-inch thickness, and cut into 1-inch-square dumplings.
3. Remove chicken from bone; return chicken to chicken stock.
4. Bring stock to a boil; add dumplings. Cover, reduce heat, and simmer 8 to 10 minutes or until dumplings are done.

Yield: 6 servings

CHICKEN FLORENTINE WITH MUSHROOM SAUCE

Exchanges: 1 Starch, 3 Lean Meat

Serving Size: ½ recipe	**Calories:** 214
Carbohydrate: 16 gm	**Fiber:** 4 gm
Protein: 24 gm	**Sodium:** 594 mg
Fat: 7 gm	**Cholesterol:** 43 mg

INGREDIENTS:

2 (3-ounce) skinned, boned chicken breast halves
¼ cup chopped onion
Vegetable cooking spray
1 (10-ounce) package frozen chopped spinach, thawed
2 tablespoons shredded reduced-fat Swiss cheese
⅛ teaspoon ground nutmeg
½ cup sliced fresh mushrooms
½ cup skim milk
½ cup water
1 tablespoon reduced-calorie margarine, melted
½ teaspoon chicken-flavored bouillon granules

STEPS IN PREPARATION:

1. Place chicken between 2 sheets of heavy-duty plastic wrap, and flatten to ¼-inch thickness using a meat mallet or rolling pin. Set chicken aside.
2. Sauté onion in a large skillet coated with cooking spray. Remove from heat, and stir in spinach, cheese, and nutmeg.
3. Divide spinach mixture in half, and shape into mounds. Transfer mounds to an 11- x 7- x 2-inch baking dish coated with cooking spray. Top each portion with a chicken breast half. Bake at 350° for 25 minutes or until chicken is done.
4. Place mushrooms in skillet. Stir in milk and remaining ingredients, and bring to a boil; boil 6 minutes or until liquid is reduced and thickened, stirring frequently. Spoon sauce evenly over chicken, and serve warm.

Yield: 2 servings

SPINACH-CHICKEN ROLLS

Exchanges: 2 Lean Meat, 1 Vegetable

Serving Size: 1 chicken roll
Carbohydrate: 8 gm
Protein: 14 gm
Fat: 2 gm

Calories: 108
Fiber: 2 gm
Sodium: 276 mg
Cholesterol: 30 mg

INGREDIENTS:

1 small onion, chopped
¼ pound fresh mushrooms, chopped
Vegetable cooking spray
1 (10-ounce) package frozen chopped spinach, thawed
2 tablespoons grated Parmesan cheese
1 tablespoon chili sauce
½ teaspoon dried whole basil
¼ teaspoon salt

8 (3-ounce) skinned, boned chicken breast halves
1 (16-ounce) can whole tomatoes, drained and chopped
⅓ cup finely chopped onion
½ teaspoon dried Italian seasoning
¼ teaspoon pepper
1 clove garlic, crushed
2 tablespoons tomato sauce

STEPS IN PREPARATION:

1. Combine 1 chopped onion and mushrooms in a shallow 2-quart casserole coated with cooking spray. Cover and microwave at HIGH 4 minutes; drain.
2. Place spinach on paper towels, and squeeze until barely moist. Add spinach and next 4 ingredients to onion mixture.
3. Place chicken between 2 sheets of heavy-duty plastic wrap; flatten to ¼-inch thickness using a meat mallet. Place ¼ cup spinach mixture in center of each chicken piece. Roll up lengthwise; secure with wooden picks. Place in casserole coated with cooking spray.
4. Combine tomato and next 4 ingredients; spoon over chicken. Cover and microwave at HIGH 12 minutes, rotating dish after 5 minutes and rearranging rolls so that uncooked portions are to outside of dish.
5. Transfer chicken to a warm platter. Stir 2 tablespoons tomato sauce into liquid in dish. Cover and microwave at HIGH 2 minutes. Spoon over chicken.

Yield: 8 servings

HONEY-MUSTARD CHICKEN NUGGETS

Exchanges: ½ Starch, 3½ Lean Meat

Serving Size: ¼ recipe
Carbohydrate: 6 gm
Protein: 27 gm
Fat: 4 gm

Calories: 169
Fiber: trace
Sodium: 239 mg
Cholesterol: 72 mg

INGREDIENTS:

1 teaspoon ground coriander
⅛ teaspoon salt
⅛ teaspoon pepper
1 pound unbreaded chicken
  breast nuggets
Vegetable cooking spray

¼ cup chopped shallots
1 large clove garlic, minced
½ cup canned low-sodium
  chicken broth, undiluted
3 tablespoons honey mustard

STEPS IN PREPARATION:

1. Combine first 3 ingredients; stir well. Add chicken, tossing to coat.
2. Coat a large nonstick skillet with cooking spray; place over medium-high heat until hot. Add shallots and garlic; sauté 1 minute. Add chicken, and cook 10 minutes or until chicken is tender, stirring frequently. Remove chicken from skillet; drain on paper towels. Wipe drippings from skillet with a paper towel.
3. Add broth and honey mustard to skillet; cook over medium heat, stirring constantly, 3 minutes or until thickened and bubbly. Add chicken; cook until thoroughly heated.

Yield: 4 servings

TURKEY HASH

Exchanges: 1 Starch, 1 Medium-Fat Meat

Serving Size: ½ cup	**Calories:** 145
Carbohydrate: 15 gm	**Fiber:** 2 gm
Protein: 11 gm	**Sodium:** 503 mg
Fat: 5 gm	**Cholesterol:** 26 mg

INGREDIENTS:

¼ cup chopped onion
2 teaspoons reduced-calorie margarine, melted
1½ cups diced cooked potatoes
1 cup diced cooked turkey breast
⅔ cup cooked English peas

1 (10¾-ounce) can cream of celery soup, undiluted
Vegetable cooking spray
¼ cup (1 ounce) shredded low-fat process American cheese
¼ teaspoon paprika

STEPS IN PREPARATION:

1. Sauté onion in margarine in a nonstick skillet until tender. Add potato and next 3 ingredients.
2. Place mixture in a 1-quart casserole coated with cooking spray. Top with shredded cheese and paprika. Bake at 350° for 30 minutes or until thoroughly heated.

Yield: 6 servings

Store fresh uncooked turkey in its original package for up to three days in the refrigerator. If you don't plan to cook it within that time, freeze it as soon as possible to maintain optimum flavor. You can freeze turkey for up to three months.

TURKEY-STUFFED TOMATOES

Exchanges: 2 Lean Meat, 2 Vegetable

Serving Size: 1 stuffed tomato
Carbohydrate: 11 gm
Protein: 17 gm
Fat: 3 gm

Calories: 134
Fiber: 2 gm
Sodium: 433 mg
Cholesterol: 35 mg

INGREDIENTS:

6 medium tomatoes
½ teaspoon salt
1 cup skim milk
1 tablespoon all-purpose
   flour
1¾ cups chopped cooked
   turkey breast

½ cup chopped celery
¼ cup chopped green onions
¼ cup (1 ounce) shredded
   low-fat process American
   cheese
½ teaspoon salt
¼ teaspoon pepper

STEPS IN PREPARATION:

1. Cut tops from tomatoes; scoop out pulp, leaving shells intact. Reserve pulp for other uses. Sprinkle inside of tomato shells with ½ teaspoon salt, and invert on paper towels to drain.
2. Combine milk and flour in a small saucepan, stirring to blend. Bring to a boil; reduce heat to low, and cook, stirring constantly, until smooth and thickened.
3. Stir in turkey, celery, onions, and cheese. Sprinkle with remaining ½ teaspoon salt and pepper.
4. Spoon turkey mixture into tomato shells, and place shells in a 13- x 9- x 2-inch baking dish. Bake at 375° for 15 to 20 minutes or until thoroughly heated.

Yield: 6 servings

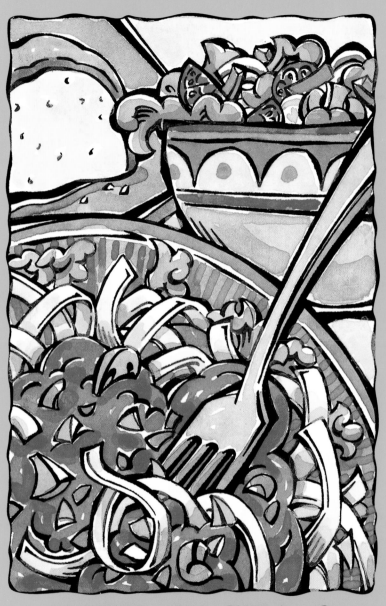

RICE, PASTA & STARCHY VEGETABLES

BAKED RICE

Exchanges: 1 Starch

Serving Size: ⅓ cup	**Calories:** 98
Carbohydrate: 19 gm	**Fiber:** 0 gm
Protein: 3 gm	**Sodium:** 473 mg
Fat: 1 gm	**Cholesterol:** 1 mg

INGREDIENTS:

1 cup long-grain rice, uncooked
Vegetable cooking spray
1 (10½-ounce) can beef
  consommé, undiluted

1 (10½-ounce) can onion soup
  in beef stock, undiluted

STEPS IN PREPARATION:

1. Place rice in a 1-quart casserole coated with cooking spray.
2. Pour consommé and soup over rice; stir well.
3. Cover and bake at 350° for 1 hour, stirring occasionally.

Yield: 9 servings

Increase the flavor of rice without adding a lot of
fat or calories by cooking it in chicken broth, beef
broth, or consommé. You can also use orange juice
or apple juice as the cooking liquid to add zest to
rice. Be sure to count the juice in your meal plan.

BAKED CHEESE AND RICE

Exchanges: 1 Starch, ½ Medium-Fat Meat

Serving Size: ⅓ cup
Carbohydrate: 19 gm
Protein: 6 gm
Fat: 3 gm

Calories: 130
Fiber: 0 gm
Sodium: 560 mg
Cholesterol: 9 mg

INGREDIENTS:

¾ cup skim milk
1 cup (4 ounces) shredded
   low-fat process American
   cheese
1 teaspoon reduced-calorie
   margarine
½ teaspoon Worcestershire
   sauce

¼ teaspoon salt
Dash of pepper
2 cups cooked long-grain rice
   (cooked without salt or fat)
Vegetable cooking spray
Dash of paprika

STEPS IN PREPARATION:

1. Combine milk and cheese in a small saucepan; cook over low heat, stirring constantly, until cheese melts.
2. Add margarine and next 3 ingredients; stir well. Add rice, and stir.
3. Spoon mixture into a 1-quart baking dish coated with cooking spray; sprinkle with paprika. Bake at 350° for 15 minutes or until lightly browned.

Yield: 7 servings

BLACK-EYED PEAS WITH RICE

Exchanges: 1 Starch

Serving Size: ⅓ cup	**Calories:** 92
Carbohydrate: 17 gm	**Fiber:** 5 gm
Protein: 5 gm	**Sodium:** 316 mg
Fat: 1 gm	**Cholesterol:** 0 mg

INGREDIENTS:

½ cup chopped onion
2 teaspoons reduced-calorie margarine, melted
⅔ cup cooked long-grain rice (cooked without salt or fat)
¼ teaspoon salt
¼ teaspoon pepper

1 (15-ounce) can black-eyed peas, drained
1 (14½-ounce) can stewed tomatoes, undrained
Vegetable cooking spray

STEPS IN PREPARATION:

1. Sauté onion in margarine in a nonstick skillet until tender.
2. Add rice and next 4 ingredients, stirring well.
3. Spoon mixture into a 1-quart casserole coated with cooking spray. Bake at 350° for 30 minutes or until thoroughly heated.

Yield: 9 servings

Legumes, such as black-eyed peas, chick-peas, lima beans, and kidney beans, are packed with complex carbohydrates, fiber, vitamins, minerals, and protein—more protein than any other edible plant food. Legumes have no cholesterol, are very low in fat and sodium, and are inexpensive.

HAM "FRIED" RICE

Exchanges: 1 Starch, 1 Medium-Fat Meat

Serving Size: ¾ cup	**Calories:** 150
Carbohydrate: 19 gm	**Fiber:** 1 gm
Protein: 9 gm	**Sodium:** 812 mg
Fat: 4 gm	**Cholesterol:** 18 mg

INGREDIENTS:

1 cup chopped celery
½ cup chopped onion
½ cup chopped green pepper
1 tablespoon reduced-calorie margarine, melted
1½ cups diced lean cooked ham

½ teaspoon salt
1 teaspoon curry powder
Dash of garlic powder
2 cups cooked long-grain rice (cooked without salt or fat)

STEPS IN PREPARATION:

1. Sauté celery, onion, and green pepper in margarine in a large nonstick skillet.
2. Add ham and next 3 ingredients, stirring well. Stir in rice. Cook over medium heat, stirring constantly, until thoroughly heated.

Yield: 7 servings

HOLIDAY RICE

Exchanges: 1 Starch

Serving Size: ½ cup	**Calories:** 99
Carbohydrate: 19 gm	**Fiber:** 1 gm
Protein: 2 gm	**Sodium:** 496 mg
Fat: 1 gm	**Cholesterol:** 0 mg

INGREDIENTS:

½ cup chopped onion
½ cup chopped celery
½ cup chopped green pepper
2 tablespoons reduced-calorie margarine, melted
2½ cups cooked long-grain rice (cooked without salt or fat)

1 cup cooked chopped broccoli
2 tablespoons chopped fresh parsley
1 teaspoon salt
Vegetable cooking spray
Fresh parsley sprigs (optional)

STEPS IN PREPARATION:

1. Sauté first 3 ingredients in margarine in a nonstick skillet.
2. Add rice, broccoli, chopped parsley, and salt; stir well.
3. Spoon mixture into a warm 5-cup ring mold coated with cooking spray, and invert onto a serving platter.
4. Garnish with parsley sprigs, if desired.

Yield: 9 servings

MEXICAN RICE

Exchanges: 1 Starch

Serving Size: ⅓ cup	**Calories:** 94
Carbohydrate: 19 gm	**Fiber:** 1 gm
Protein: 2 gm	**Sodium:** 485 mg
Fat: 1 gm	**Cholesterol:** 0 mg

INGREDIENTS:

⅔ cup chopped onion
1 tablespoon reduced-calorie margarine, melted
1 cup long-grain rice, uncooked
1 cup chopped green pepper

1 teaspoon salt
1 teaspoon chili powder
1 (8-ounce) can whole tomatoes, chopped
2 cups water

STEPS IN PREPARATION:

1. Sauté onion in margarine in a nonstick skillet until tender.
2. Stir in rice and next 4 ingredients; add water.
3. Bring to boil; reduce heat, cover, and simmer 20 minutes or until rice is tender and liquid is absorbed.

Yield: 10 servings

To cook the perfect pot of rice, remember that cooking times vary with brands and the amount of liquid recommended by each. Follow the package directions for each brand for best results. These directions usually indicate how to make rice firmer or softer to suit personal taste. You can interchange most kinds of rice in different recipes by making minor adjustments.

HINT-OF-SPICE RICE

Exchanges: 1½ Starch, 1 Fat

Serving Size: ½ cup
Carbohyrate: 25 gm
Protein: 4 gm
Fat: 4 gm

Calories: 143
Fiber: 2 gm
Sodium: 143 mg
Cholesterol: 0 mg

INGREDIENTS:

1½ cups canned low-sodium
  chicken broth, undiluted
¾ cup long-grain brown rice,
  uncooked
1 teaspoon grated orange
  rind

¼ teaspoon salt
¼ teaspoon ground ginger
¼ teaspoon ground cinnamon
1 medium orange, peeled and
  sectioned
¼ cup sliced almonds, toasted

STEPS IN PREPARATION:

1. Combine first 6 ingredients in a large saucepan; bring to a boil.
   Cover, reduce heat, and simmer 30 minutes or until rice is tender
   and liquid is absorbed.
2. Gently stir in orange sections and almonds.

Yield: 5 servings

PARSLIED RICE

Exchanges: 1 Starch, 1 Medium-Fat Meat

Serving Size: ½ cup
Carbohydrate: 17 gm
Protein: 11 gm
Fat: 7 gm

Calories: 177
Fiber: 1 gm
Sodium: 642 mg
Cholesterol: 39 mg

INGREDIENTS:

- 2 green onions, chopped
- ½ clove garlic, minced
- 3 tablespoons reduced-calorie margarine, melted
- 2 cups cooked long-grain rice (cooked without salt or fat)
- 2 cups skim milk
- 2 cups (8 ounces) shredded low-fat process American cheese
- 1 cup chopped fresh parsley
- ½ teaspoon salt
- 1 egg, lightly beaten
- Vegetable cooking spray

STEPS IN PREPARATION:

1. Sauté onions and garlic in margarine in a nonstick skillet until tender.
2. Combine onion mixture, rice, and next 5 ingredients, stirring well.
3. Spoon mixture into a 1½-quart casserole coated with cooking spray. Bake at 350° for 45 minutes or until thoroughly heated.

Yield: 8 servings

WILD RICE CASSEROLE

Exchanges: 1 Starch

Serving Size: ½ cup	**Calories:** 69
Carbohydrate: 10 gm	**Fiber:** 1 gm
Protein: 2 gm	**Sodium:** 374 mg
Fat: 2 gm	**Cholesterol:** trace

INGREDIENTS:

- 1 (10-ounce) package brown and wild rice mix
- 1 teaspoon salt
- 1 medium onion, minced
- 1 medium-size green pepper, chopped
- 2 tablespoons reduced-calorie margarine, melted
- ½ cup skim milk
- ½ (10¾-ounce) can cream of mushroom soup, undiluted
- 1 (4-ounce) jar whole pimiento, drained and minced
- Vegetable cooking spray

STEPS IN PREPARATION:

1. Cook rice according to package directions, using 1 teaspoon salt. Set aside.
2. Sauté onion and green pepper in margarine in a nonstick skillet until tender.
3. Combine rice, onion mixture, milk, soup, and pimiento, stirring well. Spoon into a 1½-quart casserole coated with cooking spray. Bake at 350° for 30 minutes or until thoroughly heated.

Yield: 10 servings

VEGETABLE-RICE CASSEROLE

Exchanges: 2 Starch

Serving Size: ½ cup	**Calories:** 147
Carbohydrate: 28 gm	**Fiber:** 4 gm
Protein: 5 gm	**Sodium:** 582 mg
Fat: 2 gm	**Cholesterol:** trace

INGREDIENTS:

2 teaspoons vegetable oil
2 cups chopped cauliflower
2 cups chopped broccoli
1 cup chopped onion, divided
2 medium-size green peppers, cut into strips
2 cloves garlic, chopped
½ teaspoon dried thyme
1 tablespoon chicken-flavored bouillon granules
3 cups hot water
1½ cups brown rice, uncooked
3 tablespoons reduced-sodium soy sauce

STEPS IN PREPARATION:

1. Place oil in a large skillet; add cauliflower, broccoli, ½ cup onion, green pepper, and garlic. Sauté 5 minutes or until tender. Stir in thyme. Remove from heat, and set aside.
2. Dissolve bouillon granules in hot water in a 2-quart casserole. Stir in remaining ½ cup onion, rice, and soy sauce. Cover and bake at 350° for 20 minutes.
3. Remove casserole from oven, and stir in vegetable mixture. Cover and bake 10 to 15 minutes or until liquid is absorbed.

Yield: 10 servings

RED BEANS AND RICE

Exchanges: 1½ Starch

Serving Size: ½ cup
Carbohydrate: 20 gm
Protein: 6 gm
Fat: trace

Calories: 106
Fiber: 5 gm
Sodium: 304 mg
Cholesterol: trace

INGREDIENTS:

Vegetable cooking spray
½ cup finely chopped celery
¼ cup chopped green onions
¼ cup chopped green pepper
1 (16-ounce) can kidney
  beans, drained
1 teaspoon beef-flavored
  bouillon granules
1 cup boiling water

1 teaspoon garlic powder
1 teaspoon dried oregano
½ teaspoon ground white
  pepper
⅛ teaspoon ground red
  pepper
1 cup cooked long-grain rice
  (cooked without salt or fat)

STEPS IN PREPARATION:

1. Coat a medium nonstick skillet with cooking spray. Place over medium heat until hot. Add celery, green onions, and green pepper; sauté 5 minutes or until tender. Stir in beans.
2. Dissolve bouillon granules in boiling water. Add to vegetable mixture. Stir in garlic powder and next 3 ingredients; bring to a boil.
3. Add cooked rice to skillet, stirring well. Cover and remove from heat. Let stand 5 minutes.

Yield: 8 servings

BLACK BEANS AND RICE

Exchanges: 3 Starch

Serving Size: 1 cup	**Calories:** 246
Carbohydrate: 48 gm	**Fiber:** 9 gm
Protein: 12 gm	**Sodium:** 240 mg
Fat: trace	**Cholesterol:** 0 mg

INGREDIENTS:

1 (16-ounce) package dried black beans
1 medium-size green pepper, chopped
¼ cup chopped onion, divided
2½ quarts water, divided
½ teaspoon dried oregano
¼ teaspoon ground cumin
2 cloves garlic, minced
3 tablespoons vinegar
1 teaspoon salt
3 cups cooked long-grain rice (cooked without salt or fat)

STEPS IN PREPARATION:

1. Sort and wash beans. Combine beans, green pepper, and 2 tablespoons onion in a large Dutch oven. Cover with 6 cups of water, and soak overnight.
2. Add remaining 4 cups water to Dutch oven; cover and bring to a boil. Reduce heat, and simmer 2½ hours or until beans are tender.
3. Combine remaining 2 tablespoons onion, oregano, cumin, and garlic in a small bowl; mash mixture, using a fork. Stir in vinegar.
4. Add vinegar mixture and salt to beans. Simmer, uncovered, an additional 20 minutes. Serve over ⅓-cup portions of cooked rice.

Yield: 9 servings

MACARONI AND CHEESE

Exchanges: 1 Starch, 1 Medium-Fat Meat

Serving Size: ½ cup
Carbohydrate: 22 gm
Protein: 8 gm
Fat: 4 gm

Calories: 160
Fiber: 1 gm
Sodium: 547 mg
Cholesterol: 9 mg

INGREDIENTS:

1½ tablespoons all-purpose flour
1½ cups skim milk, divided
1½ tablespoons reduced-calorie margarine
½ teaspoon salt
¾ cup (3 ounces) shredded low-fat process American cheese

2 cups cooked macaroni (cooked without salt or fat)
Vegetable cooking spray
¼ cup soft breadcrumbs

STEPS IN PREPARATION:

1. Combine flour and ¼ cup milk in a saucepan; stir until smooth. Add remaining 1¼ cups milk and margarine; stir well. Cook over medium heat, stirring constantly, until thickened and bubbly. Remove from heat, and add salt.
2. Add cheese, and cook over low heat, stirring constantly, until cheese melts. Remove from heat.
3. Alternate layers of macaroni and cheese sauce in a 1-quart casserole coated with cooking spray; top with breadcrumbs. Bake at 375° until mixture is bubbly and lightly browned.

Yield: 6 servings

FETTUCCINE ALFREDO

Exchanges: 2 Starch, 1 Fat

Serving Size: ½ cup	**Calories:** 187
Carbohydrate: 29 gm	**Fiber:** 2 gm
Protein: 7 gm	**Sodium:** 114 mg
Fat: 4 gm	**Cholesterol:** 39 mg

INGREDIENTS:

12 ounces fettuccine, uncooked
3 tablespoons reduced-calorie margarine
1 tablespoon all-purpose flour
½ cup skim milk
¼ cup grated Parmesan cheese

STEPS IN PREPARATION:

1. Cook fettuccine according to package directions, omitting salt and fat. Drain well; place in a large bowl, and keep warm.
2. Melt margarine in a medium saucepan over low heat; add flour. Cook, stirring constantly, 3 to 4 minutes or until smooth.
3. Add milk to flour mixture, and place over medium heat. Cook, stirring constantly, until mixture is thickened and bubbly.
4. Reduce heat to low, and stir in cheese. Cook, stirring constantly, until cheese melts and sauce is smooth.
5. Pour sauce over fettuccine, and toss gently to coat. Serve immediately.

Yield: 8 servings

FRESH BROCCOLI AND NOODLES

Exchanges: 1 Starch, ½ Fat

Serving Size: ½ cup
Carbohydrate: 13 gm
Protein: 4 gm
Fat: 3 gm

Calories: 89
Fiber: 4 gm
Sodium: 105 mg
Cholesterol: 9 mg

INGREDIENTS:

3 ounces medium egg noodles, uncooked
Vegetable cooking spray
3 cups broccoli flowerets
2 cups sliced fresh mushrooms
¼ cup chopped onion

¼ teaspoon garlic powder
¼ teaspoon coarsely ground black pepper
⅛ teaspoon salt
3 tablespoons reduced-calorie margarine

STEPS IN PREPARATION:

1. Cook noodles according to package directions, omitting salt and fat; drain and set aside.
2. Coat a wok or large nonstick skillet with cooking spray. Heat at medium-high (375°) for 2 minutes. Add broccoli, mushrooms, and onion; stir-fry 4 minutes or until broccoli is tender.
3. Add garlic powder, pepper, and salt to wok. Stir in noodles and margarine; cook over medium-high heat, stirring gently, until thoroughly heated.

Yield: 8 servings

PARSLIED NOODLES

Exchanges: 1 Starch, ½ Fat

Serving Size: ⅓ cup
Carbohydrate: 13 gm
Protein: 3 gm
Fat: 3 gm

Calories: 94
Fiber: 1 gm
Sodium: 164 mg
Cholesterol: 17 mg

INGREDIENTS:

6 ounces medium egg noodles, uncooked
¼ cup reduced-calorie margarine, melted
2 tablespoons chopped fresh parsley

Dash of garlic powder
2 tablespoons grated Parmesan cheese

STEPS IN PREPARATION:

1. Cook noodles according to package directions, omitting salt and fat; drain well. Pour margarine over noodles.
2. Add parsley and garlic powder; toss gently to coat. Sprinkle with cheese.

Yield: 9 servings

Dried pasta can be kept almost indefinitely if you store it in an airtight container in a cool, dry place. Fresh pasta is highly perishable and should be kept in an airtight container in the refrigerator and used within a week.

CREAMY LINGUINE

Exchanges: 1 Starch, ½ Fat

Serving Size: ½ cup
Carbohydrate: 14 gm
Protein: 5 gm
Fat: 2 gm

Calories: 100
Fiber: 1 gm
Sodium: 116 mg
Cholesterol: 42 mg

INGREDIENTS:

2 ounces thin egg noodles, uncooked
2 ounces spinach linguine, uncooked
3 tablespoons skim milk
1 egg, lightly beaten
¼ cup grated Parmesan cheese
1 tablespoon sliced pimiento

STEPS IN PREPARATION:

1. Cook pastas according to package directions, omitting salt and fat. Drain well; place in a large bowl, and keep warm.
2. Combine milk and egg in a small saucepan; cook over low heat 2 minutes, stirring frequently with a wire whisk. Stir in cheese and pimiento. Remove from heat.
3. Pour cheese mixture over pasta, and toss gently to coat. Serve immediately.

Yield: 6 servings

VEGETABLES AND PASTA IN CHEESE SAUCE

Exchanges: 1 Starch

Serving Size: ½ cup	**Calories:** 70
Carbohydrate: 10 gm	**Fiber:** 2 gm
Protein: 4 gm	**Sodium:** 177 mg
Fat: 1 gm	**Cholesterol:** 4 mg

INGREDIENTS:

2 cups cauliflower flowerets
2 cups diagonally sliced carrot
¼ cup minced onion
2 teaspoons reduced-calorie margarine, melted
1 tablespoon all-purpose flour
1 cup skim milk

½ cup (2 ounces) shredded reduced-fat Cheddar cheese
¼ teaspoon Worcestershire sauce
⅛ teaspoon salt
⅛ teaspoon pepper
½ cup cooked corkscrew or shell macaroni (cooked without salt or fat)

STEPS IN PREPARATION:

1. Combine cauliflower and carrot in a medium saucepan; add water to cover. Cover and bring to a boil. Reduce heat, and simmer 15 minutes or until vegetables are tender. Drain well; set aside, and keep warm.
2. Sauté onion in margarine in saucepan 2 minutes or until tender. Add flour, stirring well; cook, stirring constantly, 1 minute. Gradually add milk; cook over medium heat, stirring constantly, until mixture is thickened and bubbly.
3. Reduce heat to low, and add cheese and next 3 ingredients. Cook, stirring constantly, until cheese melts.
4. Add vegetables and pasta to cheese sauce in saucepan, stirring gently to coat vegetables and pasta. Cook over low heat until mixture is thoroughly heated, stirring gently.

Yield: 9 servings

VERMICELLI WITH TOMATO SAUCE

Exchanges: 1 Starch, 1½ Vegetable

Serving Size: 1 cup
Carbohydrate: 25 gm
Protein: 4 gm
Fat: 1 gm

Calories: 123
Fiber: 2 gm
Sodium: 286 mg
Cholesterol: 0 mg

INGREDIENTS:

½ cup chopped onion
1 teaspoon reduced-calorie margarine, melted
3 cups peeled, chopped tomato
1 teaspoon paprika

½ teaspoon salt
½ teaspoon dried basil
½ teaspoon dried oregano
⅛ teaspoon pepper
3 cups cooked vermicelli (cooked without salt or fat)

STEPS IN PREPARATION:

1. Sauté onion in margarine in a nonstick skillet.
2. Add tomato and next 5 ingredients; cover and simmer 5 minutes, stirring occasionally.
3. Remove from heat, and spoon over ½-cup portions of pasta.

Yield: 6 servings

Vermicelli is very thin pasta. Substitute thin spaghetti or angel hair pasta if vermicelli is not available.

LIMA BEANS DELUXE

Exchanges: 1 Starch, 1 Lean Meat

Serving Size: ½ cup	**Calories:** 115
Carbohydrate: 16 gm	**Fiber:** 3 gm
Protein: 7 gm	**Sodium:** 450 mg
Fat: 3 gm	**Cholesterol:** 6 mg

INGREDIENTS:

1 (10-ounce) package frozen lima beans
1 tablespoon reduced-calorie margarine
1 tablespoon all-purpose flour
1 cup skim milk
½ teaspoon salt
⅛ teaspoon pepper
½ cup (2 ounces) shredded reduced-fat Cheddar cheese
2 tablespoons reduced-calorie ketchup
2 (4-ounce) jars diced pimiento, drained
Vegetable cooking spray

STEPS IN PREPARATION:

1. Cook beans according to package directions, omitting salt and fat. Drain and set aside.
2. Melt margarine in a medium saucepan over low heat; add flour, stirring until smooth. Cook, stirring constantly, 1 minute. Gradually add milk; cook over medium heat, stirring constantly, until thickened and bubbly. Stir in salt and pepper. Remove from heat.
3. Add beans, cheese, ketchup, and pimiento to sauce; stir well. Spoon into a 1½-quart casserole coated with cooking spray. Bake at 375° for 30 minutes or until thoroughly heated.

Yield: 6 servings

ROASTED CORN ON THE COB

Exchanges: 1 Starch, ½ Fat

Serving Size: ½ ear	**Calories:** 83
Carbohydrate: 16 gm	**Fiber:** 2 gm
Protein: 2 gm	**Sodium:** 123 mg
Fat: 3 gm	**Cholesterol:** 0 mg

INGREDIENTS:

2 (8-inch) ears fresh corn	Dash of salt
4 teaspoons reduced-calorie margarine	Dash of pepper

STEPS IN PREPARATION:

1. Turn back corn husks, and remove silk.
2. Spread margarine evenly on corn; sprinkle with salt and pepper.
3. Pull husks back up, tying tightly.
4. Place corn on grill rack. Grill over hot coals (400° to 500°), uncovered, for 30 minutes, turning frequently.
5. To serve, remove ears from husks, and cut each in half.

Yield: 4 servings

SKILLET CORN

Exchanges: 1 Starch

Serving Size: ⅓ cup
Carbohydrate: 12 gm
Protein: 2 gm
Fat: 1 gm

Calories: 58
Fiber: 2 gm
Sodium: 391 mg
Cholesterol: 0 mg

INGREDIENTS:

10 ears fresh corn (about 2 cups cut corn)
½ cup skim milk
1 teaspoon salt
⅛ teaspoon pepper
1 tablespoon reduced-calorie margarine

STEPS IN PREPARATION:

1. Shuck corn, and remove silk from ears. Cut kernels from cobs. Scrape cobs gently with back of knife to get juice.
2. Add milk, salt, and pepper to corn, and stir.
3. Melt margarine in a heavy skillet. Pour corn mixture into skillet. Simmer until tender, stirring frequently.

Yield: 6 servings

Use fresh corn, green beans, and peas as soon as possible because their sweet taste diminishes with the length of storage as their sugar content turns to starch. Store these vegetables, unwashed, in plastic bags in the refrigerator for short periods of time only.

MEXICAN CORN

Exchanges: 1 Starch

Serving Size: ⅓ cup
Carbohydrate: 12 gm
Protein: 2 gm
Fat: 2 gm

Calories: 63
Fiber: 2 gm
Sodium: 349 mg
Cholesterol: 0 mg

INGREDIENTS:

2 cups canned whole kernel corn, drained
½ cup diced onion
¼ cup chopped green pepper
¼ cup chopped sweet red pepper

2 tablespoons reduced-calorie margarine, melted
1 teaspoon salt
¼ teaspoon dried oregano
¼ teaspoon ground allspice
1 cup peeled, diced tomato

STEPS IN PREPARATION:

1. Combine first 8 ingredients in a large nonstick skillet. Cover and cook over medium heat 7 minutes, stirring occasionally.
2. Add tomato; cook, uncovered, 2 minutes or until thoroughly heated.

Yield: 7 servings

CORN CUSTARD

Exchanges: 1 Starch, 1 Fat

Serving Size: ⅓ cup
Carbohydrate: 13 gm
Protein: 4 gm
Fat: 4 gm

Calories: 98
Fiber: 2 gm
Sodium: 343 mg
Cholesterol: 64 mg

INGREDIENTS:

1 (16-ounce) can cream-style corn
1 tablespoon chopped parsley
½ teaspoon onion salt
2 eggs, lightly beaten
Vegetable cooking spray

STEPS IN PREPARATION:

1. Combine first 4 ingredients in a medium bowl, stirring well.
2. Spoon mixture into a 1-quart casserole coated with cooking spray. Place casserole in a pan of warm water. Bake at 325° for 1¼ hours or until set. Serve warm.

Yield: 6 servings

If you want to reduce sodium, use canned no-salt-added cream-style corn instead of the regular product in this recipe and others.

CORN PUDDING

Exchanges: 1 Starch

Serving Size: ¼ cup
Carbohydrate: 10 gm
Protein: 4 gm
Fat: 2 gm

Calories: 62
Fiber: 1 gm
Sodium: 295 mg
Cholesterol: 47 mg

INGREDIENTS:

2 cups canned whole kernel
  corn, drained
1 cup skim milk
Sugar substitute to equal 1
  teaspoon sugar*
½ teaspoon salt

¼ teaspoon pepper
⅛ teaspoon ground allspice
2 eggs, well beaten
Vegetable cooking spray

STEPS IN PREPARATION:

1. Combine first 7 ingredients in a medium bowl, stirring well.
2. Spoon mixture into a 1-quart casserole coated with cooking spray.
   Bake at 350° for 60 to 70 minutes or until a knife inserted into
   center of pudding comes out clean. Serve warm.

Yield: 8 servings

*See the sugar substitution chart on page 354.

HASH BROWN POTATOES

Exchanges: 1 Starch

Serving Size: ½ cup
Carbohydrate: 16 gm
Protein: 1 gm
Fat: trace

Calories: 67
Fiber: 1 gm
Sodium: 270 mg
Cholesterol: 0 mg

INGREDIENTS:

Vegetable cooking spray
2 cups diced potato
½ teaspoon salt

¼ teaspoon pepper
¼ cup green onions (optional)

STEPS IN PREPARATION:

1. Coat a nonstick skillet with cooking spray. Place potato, salt, and pepper in skillet; cook over medium-high heat, stirring constantly, 2 minutes.
2. Reduce heat, and add onions, if desired; cook 30 minutes or until potato is tender, stirring occasionally.

Yield: 4 servings

Always store potatoes and onions in a well-ventilated cool, dark place to prevent them from sprouting. But don't store potatoes and onions together—the onions will absorb moisture from the potatoes, causing the onions to spoil faster.

HERBED NEW POTATOES

Exhanges: 1 Starch

Serving Size: 1 potato
Carbohydrate: 22 gm
Protein: 2 gm
Fat: 1 gm

Calories: 100
Fiber: 2 gm
Sodium: 112 mg
Cholesterol: 0 mg

INGREDIENTS:

6 small new potatoes
1 tablespoon minced fresh parsley
2 teaspoons reduced-calorie margarine

¼ teaspoon salt
Dash of pepper

STEPS IN PREPARATION:

1. Cook potatoes, covered, in boiling water to cover 20 minutes or until tender. Drain and peel potatoes.
2. Combine parsley and remaining ingredients; add to potatoes, tossing to coat.

Yield: 6 servings

POTATO CASSEROLE

Exchanges: 1 Starch, ½ Fat

Serving Size: ½ cup
Carbohydrate: 16 gm
Protein: 2 gm
Fat: 3 gm

Calories: 94
Fiber: 1 gm
Sodium: 445 mg
Cholesterol: 0 mg

INGREDIENTS:

4 medium baking potatoes,
   peeled and sliced
2 tablespoons chopped green
   pepper
2 tablespoons minced onion

½ teaspoon salt
⅛ teaspoon pepper
1 (10¾-ounce) can cream of
   mushroom soup, undiluted
Vegetable cooking spray

STEPS IN PREPARATION:

1. Combine first 6 ingredients in a medium bowl.
2. Spoon mixture into a 1-quart casserole coated with cooking spray.
   Bake at 350° for 1 to 1½ hours or until potato is tender.

Yield: 8 servings

Potatoes are practically fat-free and are a good
source of vitamins, minerals, and fiber. It's addi-
tions such as butter and sour cream that can make
potatoes fattening. Instead, try topping your potato
with nonfat yogurt or sour cream, low-fat Ranch
salad dressing, low-fat shredded cheese, vegetables, or salsa.

TWICE-BAKED POTATOES
Exchanges: 1 Starch

Serving Size: ½ potato	**Calories:** 74
Carbohydrate: 14 gm	**Fiber:** 1 gm
Protein: 3 gm	**Sodium:** 75 mg
Fat: trace	**Cholesterol:** 2 mg

INGREDIENTS:

4 small baking potatoes
½ cup skim milk
½ cup plain nonfat
  yogurt

¼ cup (1 ounce) shredded
  low-fat process American
  cheese
½ teaspoon paprika

STEPS IN PREPARATION:

1. Wash potatoes, and pat dry; prick each potato several times with a fork. Arrange potatoes end to end and 1 inch apart in a circle on paper towels in microwave oven. Microwave at HIGH 12 minutes, turning and rearranging potatoes after 6 minutes. Let potatoes stand 5 minutes.
2. Cut potatoes in half lengthwise. Scoop out pulp, leaving shells intact. Set shells aside.
3. Mash pulp in a large bowl, using a fork or potato masher. Add milk and yogurt; beat at low speed of an electric mixer until smooth and well blended. Spoon potato mixture into shells, and place on a microwave-safe serving platter.
4. Top stuffed potatoes evenly with cheese, and sprinkle with paprika. Microwave at HIGH 30 seconds or until cheese melts. Serve immediately.

Yield: 8 servings

SCALLOPED POTATOES

Exchanges: 1 Starch

Serving Size: ½ cup	**Calories:** 82
Carbohydrate: 17 gm	**Fiber:** 1 gm
Protein: 3 gm	**Sodium:** 144 mg
Fat: 1 gm	**Cholesterol:** trace

INGREDIENTS:

1 clove garlic, minced
1 tablespoon reduced-calorie margarine, melted
1 tablespoon cornstarch
½ teaspoon salt
⅛ teaspoon pepper
1½ cups skim milk
1½ pounds round red potatoes, peeled and thinly sliced
¼ cup chopped onion
¼ cup chopped fresh parsley
Vegetable cooking spray

STEPS IN PREPARATION:

1. Sauté garlic in margarine in a small saucepan until tender. Stir in cornstarch, salt, and pepper.
2. Add milk, stirring well. Cook over medium heat, stirring constantly, 2 minutes or until mixture is thickened and bubbly. Remove sauce from heat, and set aside.
3. Arrange half each of potato, onion, and parsley in a 2-quart casserole coated with cooking spray. Top with half of sauce. Repeat layers with remaining potato, onion, parsley, and sauce.
4. Cover and bake at 350° for 45 minutes, stirring once. Uncover and bake an additional 30 minutes or until potato is tender.

Yield: 10 servings

POTATO-CHEESE CASSEROLE

Exchanges: 1 Starch, ½ Fat

Serving Size: ½ cup
Carbohydrate: 18 gm
Protein: 4 gm
Fat: 2 gm

Calories: 103
Fiber: 1 gm
Sodium: 215 mg
Cholesterol: 27 mg

INGREDIENTS:

3 cups cooked, mashed potato
(cooked without salt or fat)
1 egg, separated
½ cup (2 ounces) shredded
low-fat process American
cheese
1 tablespoon finely chopped
green onions

½ teaspoon celery salt
½ small green pepper, finely
chopped
1 egg white
Vegetable cooking spray
½ teaspoon paprika

STEPS IN PREPARATION:

1. Combine mashed potato and egg yolk, stirring until well blended.
Stir in cheese, green onions, celery salt, and green pepper.
2. Beat 2 egg whites (at room temperature) at high speed of an electric
mixer until soft peaks form. Gently fold egg whites into potato
mixture.
3. Spoon mixture into a 1½-quart casserole coated with cooking
spray. Sprinkle paprika evenly over top of casserole. Bake at 375°
for 25 to 30 minutes or until thoroughly heated.

Yield: 8 servings

SWEET POTATO CASSEROLE

Exchanges: 1½ Starch, ½ Fat

Serving Size: ⅓ cup	**Calories:** 132
Carbohydrate: 24 gm	**Fiber:** 1 gm
Protein: 3 gm	**Sodium:** 96 mg
Fat: 3 gm	**Cholesterol:** 31 mg

INGREDIENTS:

1 (18-ounce) can sweet
   potatoes, drained
1 cup granulated brown
   sugar substitute, divided
¼ cup skim milk
1 tablespoon reduced-calorie
   margarine, melted
1 teaspoon vanilla extract
1 egg
Vegetable cooking spray
1 tablespoon all-purpose flour
1 tablespoon reduced-calorie
   margarine

STEPS IN PREPARATION:

1. Combine sweet potato, ¾ cup brown sugar substitute, and next 4
   ingredients, stirring until well blended. Spoon mixture into a
   shallow baking dish coated with cooking spray.
2. Combine flour and remaining ¼ cup brown sugar substitute; cut
   in 1 tablespoon margarine until mixture is crumbly.
3. Sprinkle flour mixture over potatoes, and bake at 350° for 35
   minutes or until thoroughly heated.

Yield: 6 servings

SPICED SWEET POTATOES

Exchanges: 1 Starch, ½ Fat

Serving Size: ¼ cup
Carbohydrate: 14 gm
Protein: 1 gm
Fat: 3 gm

Calories: 86
Fiber: 2 gm
Sodium: 182 mg
Cholesterol: 0 mg

INGREDIENTS:

2 cups cooked or canned
  sliced sweet potatoes
Vegetable cooking spray
3 tablespoons granulated
  brown sugar substitute

¼ teaspoon salt
¼ teaspoon ground cinnamon
¼ teaspoon ground nutmeg
3 tablespoons reduced-calorie
  margarine

STEPS IN PREPARATION:

1. Arrange sweet potato in a 1½-quart casserole coated with cooking spray.
2. Combine sugar substitute, salt, cinnamon, and nutmeg; sprinkle over sweet potatoes. Dot with margarine. Bake at 350° for 10 to 15 minutes or until thoroughly heated.

Yield: 6 servings

Choose sweet potatoes that are firm, plump, blemish-free, and of uniform size. Store them in a cool, dry, well-ventilated place for up to two months. (Don't refrigerate them.) For longer storage, cook, mash, and then freeze sweet potatoes.

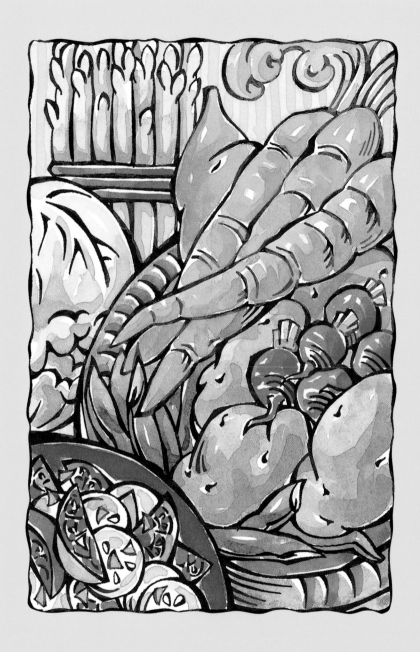

VEGETABLES

ASPARAGUS WITH BLUE CHEESE AND ALMONDS

Exchanges: 1 Vegetable

Serving Size: ⅙ recipe	**Calories:** 44
Carbohydrate: 5 gm	**Fiber:** 2 gm
Protein: 3 gm	**Sodium:** 37 mg
Fat: 2 gm	**Cholesterol:** 2 mg

INGREDIENTS:

1½ pounds fresh asparagus spears
¾ cup canned no-salt-added chicken broth, undiluted
¼ cup sliced green onions
1 teaspoon dried tarragon

12 Bibb lettuce leaves
2 tablespoons crumbled blue cheese
1½ tablespoons sliced almonds, toasted

STEPS IN PREPARATION:

1. Snap off tough ends of asparagus. Remove scales with a knife or vegetable peeler, if desired.
2. Place broth in a large skillet. Bring to a boil over medium-high heat. Add asparagus, green onions, and tarragon. Reduce heat, and simmer, uncovered, 6 to 8 minutes or until asparagus is crisp-tender. Remove asparagus from skillet, using a slotted spoon; discard broth remaining in skillet.
3. Arrange asparagus on lettuce leaves. Sprinkle with blue cheese and almonds.

Yield: 6 servings

ASPARAGUS WITH LEMON SAUCE

Exchanges: 1 Vegetable, ½ Fat

Serving Size: ½ cup
Carbohydrate: 7 gm
Protein: 1 gm
Fat: 2 gm

Calories: 49
Fiber: 1 gm
Sodium: 37 mg
Cholesterol: 31 mg

INGREDIENTS:

1 (10-ounce) package frozen asparagus spears
Sugar substitute to equal ½ cup sugar*
½ teaspoon cornstarch
1 egg

1 tablespoon reduced-calorie margarine
¼ cup lemon juice
2 teaspoons grated lemon rind

STEPS IN PREPARATION:

1. Cook asparagus according to package directions, omitting salt and fat; drain well. Transfer cooked asparagus to a serving dish, and keep warm.
2. Combine sugar substitute, cornstarch, and egg, stirring to blend. Melt margarine over low heat in a small skillet; add egg mixture. Cook over medium heat until mixture thickens.
3. Stir in lemon juice, and cook over medium heat until thickened and bubbly. Pour over asparagus, and sprinkle with lemon rind. Serve immediately.

Yield: 6 servings

*See the sugar substitution chart on page 354.

ASPARAGUS CASSEROLE

Exchanges: 1 Vegetable, ½ Fat

Serving Size: ½ cup	**Calories:** 55
Carbohydrate: 5 gm	**Fiber:** trace
Protein: 3 gm	**Sodium:** 435 mg
Fat: 2 gm	**Cholesterol:** 3 mg

INGREDIENTS:

1 (10-ounce) package frozen asparagus spears
½ cup skim milk
½ (10¾-ounce) can cream of mushroom soup, undiluted

1 (8-ounce) can sliced water chestnuts, drained
½ cup (2 ounces) shredded reduced-fat Cheddar cheese
Vegetable cooking spray

STEPS IN PREPARATION:

1. Cook asparagus according to package directions, omitting salt and fat; drain and set aside.
2. Combine milk and soup, stirring until blended. Layer half each of asparagus, soup mixture, water chestnuts, and cheese in a 1½-quart casserole coated with cooking spray.
3. Repeat layers with remaining asparagus, soup mixture, water chestnuts, and cheese. Bake at 325° for 20 minutes or until thoroughly heated.

Yield: 8 servings

PICKLED BEETS

Exchanges: 1 Vegetable

Serving Size: ½ cup	**Calories:** 32
Carbohydrate: 8 gm	**Fiber:** 2 gm
Protein: 1 gm	**Sodium:** 69 mg
Fat: trace	**Cholesterol:** 0 mg

INGREDIENTS:

1¾ cups canned sliced beets, drained
½ cup vinegar
Sugar substitute to equal 3 tablespoons sugar*

6 whole cloves
1 slice lemon
1 small onion, thinly sliced

STEPS IN PREPARATION:

1. Place beets in a shallow dish; add vinegar and next 3 ingredients.
2. Separate onion slices into rings, and add to beets.
3. Cover and chill at least 4 hours.

Yield: 6 servings

*See the sugar substitution chart on page 354.

BROCCOLI CASSEROLE

Exchanges: 3 Vegetable, 1 Fat

Serving Size: 1 cup
Carbohydrate: 15 gm
Protein: 6 gm
Fat: 5 gm

Calories: 123
Fiber: 3 gm
Sodium: 681 mg
Cholesterol: 7 mg

INGREDIENTS:

1 pound fresh broccoli
1 cup water
½ teaspoon salt
¼ cup chopped onion
¼ cup chopped celery
¼ pound fresh mushrooms, sliced
2 teaspoons reduced-calorie margarine, melted
1 (8-ounce) can sliced water chestnuts, drained

½ cup (2 ounces) shredded low-fat process American cheese, divided
½ cup skim milk
½ (10¾-ounce) can cream of mushroom soup, undiluted
⅛ teaspoon garlic powder
⅛ teaspoon pepper
Vegetable cooking spray

STEPS IN PREPARATION:

1. Trim off large leaves of broccoli; remove tough ends of lower stalks. Wash thoroughly; cut into 1-inch pieces.
2. Bring water to a boil in a large saucepan; add broccoli and salt. Cover, reduce heat, and simmer 5 minutes or until tender. Drain and set aside.
3. Sauté onion, celery, and mushrooms in margarine in saucepan until tender. Combine broccoli, sautéed vegetables, and water chestnuts in a large bowl; set aside.
4. Combine ¼ cup cheese, milk, and soup in saucepan; cook over low heat, stirring constantly, until cheese melts. Stir in garlic powder and pepper. Pour over broccoli mixture, tossing to coat.
5. Spoon mixture into a 2-quart casserole coated with cooking spray. Bake at 350° for 25 minutes; sprinkle with remaining ¼ cup cheese. Bake an additional 5 minutes or until cheese melts.

Yield: 5 servings

CHINESE BROCCOLI

Exchanges: 2 Vegetable

Serving Size: ½ cup	**Calories:** 51
Carbohydrate: 8 gm	**Fiber:** 4 gm
Protein: 4 gm	**Sodium:** 177 mg
Fat: 1 gm	**Cholesterol:** 0 mg

INGREDIENTS:

1 pound fresh broccoli
Vegetable cooking spray
1 tablespoon reduced-sodium
soy sauce

1 tablespoon sesame seeds,
toasted
1 sweet red pepper, sliced

STEPS IN PREPARATION:

1. Trim off large leaves of broccoli; remove tough ends of lower stalks. Wash thoroughly; separate into spears, and cut into ¼-inch diagonal slices.
2. Arrange broccoli in a vegetable steamer over boiling water. Cover and steam 3 to 5 minutes or until crisp-tender.
3. Coat a large nonstick skillet with cooking spray. Add soy sauce, and place over medium heat until hot. Add broccoli; cook, stirring constantly, 1 to 2 minutes or until tender.
4. Transfer broccoli to a serving dish. Sprinkle with sesame seeds, and garnish with pepper slices.

Yield: 4 servings

Broccoli is one of the best nutrition bets in the produce section. A medium-size stalk provides 100 percent of the Recommended Daily Allowance for vitamin C. Broccoli is also rich in vitamin A, high in fiber, and low in calories.

BROCCOLI AND RICE CASSEROLE

Exchanges: 1 Starch, 1 Medium-Fat Meat, 1 Vegetable

Serving Size: ¾ cup	**Calories:** 188
Carbohydrate: 24 gm	**Fiber:** 2 gm
Protein: 9 gm	**Sodium:** 996 mg
Fat: 6 gm	**Cholesterol:** 14 mg

INGREDIENTS:

1 (10-ounce) package frozen chopped broccoli
½ cup chopped onion
½ cup chopped celery
1 teaspoon reduced-calorie margarine, melted
1 cup (4 ounces) grated reduced-fat Cheddar cheese
1 (10¾-ounce) can cream of chicken soup, undiluted
1½ cups cooked long-grain rice (cooked without salt or fat)
¼ teaspoon salt
¼ teaspoon hot sauce
⅛ teaspoon pepper
Vegetable cooking spray
1 tablespoon soft breadcrumbs

STEPS IN PREPARATION:

1. Cook broccoli according to package directions, omitting salt and fat; drain well.
2. Sauté onion and celery in margarine in a nonstick skillet until tender.
3. Combine broccoli, cheese, and soup; add to onion mixture. Stir in rice and next 3 ingredients.
4. Spoon mixture into a 1½-quart casserole coated with cooking spray; top with breadcrumbs. Bake at 350° for 45 minutes or until thoroughly heated.

Yield: 6 servings

GREEN BEAN CASSEROLE

Exchanges: ½ Medium-Fat Meat, 1 Vegetable

Serving Size: ½ cup
Carbohydrate: 5 gm
Protein: 4 gm
Fat: 2 gm

Calories: 54
Fiber: 2 gm
Sodium: 365 mg
Cholesterol: 72 mg

INGREDIENTS:

1 (10-ounce) package frozen
chopped spinach, thawed
1 (9-ounce) package frozen
green beans, thawed
½ cup chopped onion
¼ cup water
1 teaspoon salt
1 teaspoon dried basil
⅛ teaspoon garlic powder

⅛ teaspoon ground nutmeg
⅛ teaspoon pepper
3 eggs, lightly beaten
Vegetable cooking spray
¼ cup (1 ounce) shredded
low-fat process American
cheese
1 teaspoon paprika

STEPS IN PREPARATION:

1. Drain spinach and green beans well. Combine spinach, beans,
   onion, and next 6 ingredients in a medium saucepan. Cover and
   simmer 10 minutes, stirring occasionally. Remove from heat.
2. Gradually stir vegetable mixture into beaten eggs; stir well.
3. Spoon mixture into a 1-quart casserole coated with cooking spray.
   Bake, uncovered, at 350° for 20 minutes or until set.
4. Sprinkle with cheese and paprika; bake 2 to 3 minutes or until
   cheese melts.

Yield: 8 servings

SPANISH GREEN BEANS

Exchanges: 1 Vegetable, ½ Fat

Serving Size: ½ cup
Carbohydrate: 10 gm
Protein: 2 gm
Fat: 2 gm

Calories: 55
Fiber: 3 gm
Sodium: 449 mg
Cholesterol: 0 mg

INGREDIENTS:

3¾ cups fresh green beans
1 onion, chopped
2 tablespoons reduced-calorie margarine, melted
1½ teaspoons salt

½ teaspoon garlic powder
¼ teaspoon black pepper
5 medium tomatoes, diced
2 medium-size green peppers, chopped

STEPS IN PREPARATION:

1. Wash beans; trim ends, and remove strings. Cut beans into 1½-inch pieces.
2. Sauté onion in margarine in a nonstick skillet until tender.
3. Add beans, salt, garlic powder, and black pepper. Cover and cook over low heat 10 minutes, stirring frequently.
4. Stir in tomato and green pepper; cover and simmer 25 to 30 minutes or until beans are tender.

Yield: 8 servings

MARINATED GREEN BEANS AND ONIONS

Exchanges: 1 Vegetable

Serving Size: ½ cup
Carbohydrate: 5 gm
Protein: 2 gm
Fat: 1 gm

Calories: 32
Fiber: 3 gm
Sodium: 998 mg
Cholesterol: 8 mg

INGREDIENTS:

2 cups canned green beans, drained
1 cup commercial no-oil Italian salad dressing
¼ teaspoon salt
⅛ teaspoon pepper
1 small onion, sliced

STEPS IN PREPARATION:

1. Combine all ingredients in a large bowl, and stir well. Cover and chill at least 8 hours.
2. Serve warm or chilled.

Yield: 4 servings

Use canned no-salt-added green beans in this recipe and others to reduce the sodium content.

COPPER PENNIES

Exchanges: 1 Starch, ½ Fat

Serving Size: ¾ cup	**Calories:** 111
Carbohydrate: 20 gm	**Fiber:** 5 gm
Protein: 3 gm	**Sodium:** 462 mg
Fat: 3 gm	**Cholesterol:** 1 mg

INGREDIENTS:

3½ cups sliced carrot
2 medium onions, sliced
2 medium-size green peppers, sliced
½ cup skim milk
½ cup commercial no-oil Italian dressing

1 tablespoon prepared mustard
1 tablespoon Worcestershire sauce
½ (10¾-ounce) can tomato soup, undiluted

STEPS IN PREPARATION:

1. Cook carrot in boiling water to cover in a medium saucepan until tender; drain and cool. Add onion and green pepper.
2. Combine milk and remaining ingredients; pour over carrot mixture.
3. Cover and chill.

Yield: 6 servings

The darker the orange color of carrots, the more vitamin A they contain.

CARROTS VICHY

Exchanges: 2 Vegetable

Serving Size: ½ cup	**Calories:** 51
Carbohydrate: 10 gm	**Fiber:** 2 gm
Protein: 7 gm	**Sodium:** 432 mg
Fat: 1 gm	**Cholesterol:** 0 mg

INGREDIENTS:

1 tablespoon reduced-calorie margarine
3 cups sliced carrot
¾ cup water
1 teaspoon salt
¼ teaspoon ground nutmeg
⅛ teaspoon pepper
¼ cup chopped fresh parsley
1 tablespoon lemon juice
Sugar substitute to equal 2 teaspoons sugar*

STEPS IN PREPARATION:

1. Place margarine in a saucepan. Add carrot and next 4 ingredients.
2. Bring to a boil; reduce heat, cover, and simmer 8 to 10 minutes or until crisp-tender.
3. Stir in parsley, lemon juice, and sugar substitute. Serve warm.

Yield: 6 servings

*See the sugar substitution chart on page 354.

EGGPLANT CREOLE

Exchanges: ½ Starch

Serving Size: ½ cup	**Calories:** 36
Carbohydrate: 9 gm	**Fiber:** 2 gm
Protein: 1 gm	**Sodium:** 410 mg
Fat: trace	**Cholesterol:** 0 mg

INGREDIENTS:

1 small onion, chopped
1 small green pepper, chopped
1 (8-ounce) can tomato sauce
1 clove garlic, minced
½ teaspoon salt
¼ teaspoon oregano
¼ teaspoon hot sauce
⅛ teaspoon pepper
1 small eggplant, peeled and diced

STEPS IN PREPARATION:

1. Combine first 8 ingredients in a nonstick skillet. Cover and cook over low heat 10 minutes.
2. Add eggplant; cover and cook 20 minutes or until eggplant is tender, stirring occasionally.

Yield: 6 servings

Eggplant flesh darkens rapidly when cut, so don't peel it until just before cooking. Rub cut surfaces with lemon or lime juice to prevent darkening.

COMPANY CAULIFLOWER CASSEROLE

Exchanges: 1 Vegetable

Serving Size: ½ cup	**Calories:** 22
Carbohydrate: 3 gm	**Fiber:** trace
Protein: 2 gm	**Sodium:** 88 mg
Fat: 1 gm	**Cholesterol:** 1 mg

INGREDIENTS:

1 medium cauliflower, cut into flowerets
Vegetable cooking spray
½ teaspoon salt
⅛ teaspoon pepper
½ cup plain low-fat yogurt

2 tablespoons (½ ounce) shredded reduced-fat Cheddar cheese
1 teaspoon sesame seeds, toasted

STEPS IN PREPARATION:

1. Arrange cauliflower in a vegetable steamer over boiling water. Cover and steam 8 minutes or until tender.
2. Place half of cauliflower in a 1-quart casserole coated with cooking spray; sprinkle with salt and pepper. Top with half each of yogurt and cheese.
3. Repeat layers with remaining cauliflower, yogurt, and cheese. Sprinkle with sesame seeds, and bake at 350° for 20 minutes or until thoroughly heated.

Yield: 10 servings

SPINACH-CHEESE CASSEROLE

Exchanges: 1 Lean Meat, 1 Vegetable

Serving Size: ½ cup
Carbohydrate: 6 gm
Protein: 9 gm
Fat: 3 gm

Calories: 81
Fiber: 1 gm
Sodium: 318 mg
Cholesterol: 7 mg

INGREDIENTS:

1 (10-ounce) package frozen chopped spinach
1 medium onion, chopped
2 teaspoons reduced-calorie margarine, melted
1 cup 1% low-fat cottage cheese

¼ cup (1 ounce) shredded low-fat process American cheese, divided
⅛ teaspoon ground nutmeg
Dash of pepper
Vegetable cooking spray

STEPS IN PREPARATION:

1. Cook spinach according to package directions, omitting salt; drain well.
2. Sauté onion in margarine in a medium nonstick skillet until tender. Add spinach, cottage cheese, 2 tablespoons shredded cheese, nutmeg, and pepper; stir well.
3. Spoon into a 1-quart casserole coated wih cooking spray. Sprinkle with remaining 2 tablespoons shredded cheese. Bake at 350° for 25 to 30 minutes or until set.

Yield: 5 servings

OKRA CREOLE
Exchanges: 1 Vegetable

Serving Size: ⅓ cup
Carbohydrate: 8 gm
Protein: 1 gm
Fat: trace

Calories: 36
Fiber: 2 gm
Sodium: 228 mg
Cholesterol: 0 mg

INGREDIENTS:

1½ cups sliced fresh okra
½ cup chopped onion
½ cup chopped celery
½ teaspoon salt
¼ teaspoon pepper
⅛ teaspoon ground oregano

1 (16-ounce) can whole tomatoes, undrained and chopped
1 (7-ounce) can whole kernel corn, undrained

STEPS IN PREPARATION:

1. Combine all ingredients in a heavy nonstick skillet. Bring mixture to a boil.
2. Reduce heat; cover and simmer 15 to 20 minutes or until okra is tender.

Yield: 11 servings

OKRA FROM THE OVEN

Exchanges: 2 Vegetable

Serving Size: ½ cup
Carbohydrate: 10 gm
Protein: 2 gm
Fat: trace

Calories: 44
Fiber: 4 gm
Sodium: 138 mg
Cholesterol: 0 mg

INGREDIENTS:

3 cups sliced fresh okra
Vegetable cooking spray
1 cup chopped tomato
1 cup chopped onion

1 cup chopped green pepper
½ teaspoon salt
⅛ teaspoon pepper

STEPS IN PREPARATION:

1. Spread okra in a 13- x 9- x 2-inch baking dish coated with cooking spray.
2. Layer tomato, onion, and green pepper over okra. Sprinkle with salt and pepper.
3. Cover and bake at 400° for 1 hour or until okra is tender, stirring occasionally.

Yield: 8 servings

Fresh okra should have firm, bright green pods less than four inches long. To store, keep it in a plastic bag in the refrigerator for up to three days.

SKILLET OKRA

Exchanges: 1 Starch

Serving Size: ½ cup
Carbohyrate: 17 gm
Protein: 3 gm
Fat: 1 gm

Calories: 77
Fiber: 3 gm
Sodium: 283 mg
Cholesterol: 0 mg

INGREDIENTS:

1½ cups sliced fresh okra
½ cup chopped onion
½ cup chopped celery
¼ cup chopped green pepper
1 (16-ounce) can whole
  tomatoes, undrained and
  chopped

1 (16-ounce) can whole-kernel
  corn, undrained

STEPS IN PREPARATION:

1. Combine all ingredients in a large nonstick skillet, stirring well.
   Cover and bring to a boil.
2. Reduce heat, and simmer 15 to 20 minutes or until vegetables are
   tender.

Yield: 8 servings

PARMESAN PEAS

Exchanges: 1 Starch

Serving Size: ½ cup
Carbohydrate: 12 gm
Protein: 5 gm
Fat: 1 gm

Calories: 72
Fiber: 4 gm
Sodium: 96 mg
Cholesterol: trace

INGREDIENTS:

2 (10-ounce) packages frozen English peas
1 tablespoon grated Parmesan cheese
1 teaspoon lemon juice
1 teaspoon reduced-calorie margarine, melted
¼ teaspoon dried Italian seasoning
⅛ teaspoon grated lemon rind

STEPS IN PREPARATION:

1. Cook peas according to package directions, omitting salt and fat; drain.
2. Add cheese and remaining ingredients; toss to coat. Serve warm.

Yield: 6 servings

DILLY SQUASH

Exchanges: 1 Vegetable

Serving Size: ½ cup	**Calories:** 27
Carbohydrate: 6 gm	**Fiber:** 2 gm
Protein: 1 gm	**Sodium:** 401 mg
Fat: trace	**Cholesterol:** 0 mg

INGREDIENTS:

3 cups sliced yellow squash
1 teaspoon minced onion
1 tablespoon chopped fresh
  parsley

½ teaspoon salt
¼ teaspoon dried dillweed
1 tablespoon dry butter
  substitute

STEPS IN PREPARATION:

1. Arrange squash and onion in a vegetable steamer over boiling water. Cover and steam 5 minutes or until tender.
2. Remove from heat, and mash squash mixture.
3. Add parsley, salt, and dillweed; toss lightly.
4. Sprinkle with butter substitute, and serve warm.

Yield: 4 servings

Check the stems of yellow squash to determine its quality. If stems are hard, dry, shriveled, or darkened, the squash is not fresh.

BAKED SQUASH WITH ROSEMARY

Exchanges: 1 Vegetable, ½ Fat

Serving Size: 1 cup	**Calories:** 54
Carbohydrate: 8 gm	**Fiber:** 2 gm
Protein: 2 gm	**Sodium:** 13 mg
Fat: 2 gm	**Cholesterol:** trace

INGREDIENTS:

2 pounds yellow squash
1 tablespoon low-sodium beef-flavored bouillon granules
1 cup hot water

1 teaspoon reduced-calorie margarine, melted
½ teaspoon dried rosemary, crushed

STEPS IN PREPARATION:

1. Cut yellow squash in half lengthwise. Place squash halves, cut side down, in a large shallow baking dish.
2. Dissolve bouillon granules in hot water, and pour bouillon around squash in baking dish. Bake, uncovered, at 350° for 20 minutes.
3. Combine margarine and rosemary, stirring well.
4. Turn squash, and baste with margarine mixture. Bake, uncovered, 15 minutes or until squash is tender.

Yield: 6 servings

SQUASH CASSEROLE

Exchanges: 1 Vegetable, ½ Fat

Serving Size: ½ cup
Carbohydrate: 4 gm
Protein: 2 gm
Fat: 2 gm

Calories: 42
Fiber: 1 gm
Sodium: 360 mg
Cholesterol: 37 mg

INGREDIENTS:

1 pound yellow squash
½ cup chopped onion
¼ cup chopped green pepper
2 tablespoons reduced-calorie mayonnaise
1 teaspoon salt
2 (4-ounce) jars diced pimiento, drained

1 egg
Vegetable cooking spray
2 tablespoons cracker crumbs
¼ cup (1 ounce) shredded reduced-fat Cheddar cheese

STEPS IN PREPARATION:

1. Cook squash in boiling water to cover in a medium saucepan 15 minutes or until tender. Drain and mash.
2. Combine onion and next 5 ingredients in a medium bowl, stirring well. Stir in squash.
3. Spoon squash mixture into a 2-quart casserole coated with cooking spray. Sprinkle with cracker crumbs.
4. Bake at 325° for 25 minutes. Top with cheese, and bake an additional 5 minutes or until cheese melts.

Yield: 8 servings

BAKED ZUCCHINI SQUASH

Exchanges: 1 Vegetable

Serving Size: 2 squash halves
Carbohydrate: 11 gm
Protein: 2 gm
Fat: 1 gm

Calories: 53
Fiber: 2 gm
Sodium: 312 mg
Cholesterol: 1 mg

INGREDIENTS:

4 small zucchini, cut in half
  lengthwise
¼ cup plain low-fat yogurt
3 tablespoons minced onion
3 tablespoons chopped green
  pepper
Sugar substitute to equal 2
  teaspoons sugar*

¼ teaspoon salt
⅛ teaspoon ground allspice
⅛ teaspoon pepper
1 tablespoon dry butter
  substitute
4 saltine crackers, crushed

STEPS IN PREPARATION:

1. Cook zucchini in boiling water to cover in a medium saucepan 5 minutes or until crisp-tender. Drain well, and set aside.
2. Scoop out zucchini pulp, and place in a bowl; reserve zucchini shells.
3. Combine pulp, yogurt, and next 6 ingredients.
4. Spoon mixture into squash shells. Sprinkle with butter substitute and cracker crumbs. Bake at 350° for 30 minutes or until thoroughly heated.

Yield: 4 servings

*See the sugar substitution chart on page 354.

SAUTÉED ZUCCHINI

Exchanges: 1 Vegetable, ½ Fat

Serving Size: ½ cup
Carbohydrate: 8 gm
Protein: 3 gm
Fat: 2 gm

Calories: 53
Fiber: 2 gm
Sodium: 274 mg
Cholesterol: 3 mg

INGREDIENTS:

½ cup chopped onion
1 tablespoon reduced-calorie margarine, melted
3½ cups sliced zucchini
1 cup sliced mushrooms
½ teaspoon salt

½ teaspoon dried thyme
¼ teaspoon pepper
¼ cup (1 ounce) shredded low-fat process American cheese

STEPS IN PREPARATION:

1. Sauté onion in margarine in a nonstick skillet until tender.
2. Add zucchini and next 4 ingredients. Cook over low heat 5 to 7 minutes or until zucchini is crisp-tender, stirring frequently.
3. Sprinkle with cheese, and serve immediately.

Yield: 6 servings

STUFFED BUTTERNUT SQUASH

Exchanges: ½ Starch

Serving Size: ½ cup	**Calories:** 55
Carbohydrate: 9 gm	**Fiber:** 2 gm
Protein: 2 gm	**Sodium:** 137 mg
Fat: 2 gm	**Cholesterol:** 1 mg

INGREDIENTS:

1 medium butternut squash
½ cup water
1 cup finely chopped apple
¼ cup chopped onion
2 teaspoons reduced-calorie margarine, melted
½ cup 1% low-fat cottage cheese

¼ teaspoon salt
⅛ teaspoon ground cinnamon
⅛ teaspoon ground ginger
⅛ teaspoon pepper
½ teaspoon apple pie spice

STEPS IN PREPARATION:

1. Cut squash in half lengthwise, and remove seeds. Place halves, cut side down, in an 11- x 7- x 2-inch baking dish. Pour water around squash, and bake at 350° for 45 minutes or until squash is tender.
2. Sauté apple and onion in margarine in a large nonstick skillet until onion is tender. Stir in cottage cheese and next 4 ingredients. Remove from heat, and set aside.
3. Carefully scoop out squash pulp, reserving shells. Chop pulp.
4. Add squash pulp to apple mixture in skillet, stirring well. Spoon mixture into squash shells, and sprinkle with apple pie spice. Bake at 375° for 15 minutes or until thoroughly heated.

Yield: 8 servings

STEWED TOMATOES

Exchanges: 1 Vegetable

Serving Size: ½ cup
Carbohydrate: 9 gm
Protein: 2 gm
Fat: 1 gm

Calories: 55
Fiber: 2 gm
Sodium: 350 mg
Cholesterol: 0 mg

INGREDIENTS:

1 tablespoon chopped green pepper
1 tablespoon chopped onion
1 tablespoon reduced-calorie margarine, melted

3 cups canned tomatoes, drained
2 slices white bread, cubed
¼ teaspoon salt
⅛ teaspoon black pepper

STEPS IN PREPARATION:

1. Sauté green pepper and onion in margarine in a medium nonstick skillet until tender.
2. Add tomato, bread, salt, and black pepper. Cook over medium heat until thoroughly heated, stirring occasionally.

Yield: 6 servings

SPINACH-STUFFED TOMATOES

Exchanges: 2 Vegetable

Serving Size: 1 stuffed tomato	**Calories:** 55
Carbohydrate: 10 gm	**Fiber:** 2 gm
Protein: 2 gm	**Sodium:** 191 mg
Fat: 1 gm	**Cholesterol:** trace

INGREDIENTS:

8 medium tomatoes
1 (10-ounce) package frozen chopped spinach, thawed
2 teaspoons reduced-calorie margarine
2 tablespoons all-purpose flour

½ teaspoon salt
½ teaspoon dry mustard
¼ teaspoon Worcestershire sauce
2 tablespoons soft breadcrumbs
Vegetable cooking spray

STEPS IN PREPARATION:

1. Cut tops from tomatoes; scoop out pulp, leaving shells intact. Chop pulp, and set aside. Invert tomato shells on paper towels; drain 10 minutes.
2. Cook spinach according to package directions, omitting salt and fat. Drain well.
3. Melt margarine in a medium saucepan over low heat; add flour, salt, mustard, and Worcestershire sauce, stirring until smooth. Cook, stirring constantly, 1 minute. Stir in tomato pulp and spinach. Remove from heat.
4. Spoon spinach mixture into tomato shells. Top with breadcrumbs, and place in a shallow baking dish coated with cooking spray. Bake at 400° for 15 minutes or until mixture is thoroughly heated and breadcrumbs are lightly browned.

Yield: 8 servings

BAKED TOMATOES

Exchanges: 1 Vegetable

Serving Size: 2 tomato halves
Carbohydrate: 11 gm
Protein: 2 gm
Fat: 1 gm

Calories: 56
Fiber: 1 gm
Sodium: 193 mg
Cholesterol: 0 mg

INGREDIENTS:

4 medium tomatoes, cut in half
Vegetable cooking spray
¼ teaspoon salt
⅛ teaspoon pepper
¼ cup soft breadcrumbs, toasted

3 tablespoons minced fresh parsley
¼ teaspoon dried thyme
¼ teaspoon dried oregano
⅛ teaspoon garlic powder
Fresh parsley sprigs (optional)

STEPS IN PREPARATION:

1. Place tomato halves, cut side up, in an 11- x 7- x 2-inch baking dish coated with cooking spray. Sprinkle with salt and pepper.
2. Combine breadcrumbs and next 4 ingredients; stir well.
3. Spoon mixture evenly over tomato halves. Bake at 350° for 12 to 15 minutes or until thoroughly heated. Garnish with parsley sprigs, if desired.

Yield: 4 servings

SCALLOPED TOMATOES

Exchanges: 1 Vegetable

Serving Size: ½ cup
Carbohydrate: 14 gm
Protein: 2 gm
Fat: 1 gm

Calories: 70
Fiber: 1 gm
Sodium: 580 mg
Cholesterol: 1 mg

INGREDIENTS:

1 (20-ounce) can tomatoes
1 beef bouillon cube
1 cup cubed white bread
2 tablespoons chopped onion
2 tablespoons chopped celery

½ teaspoon salt
2 tablespoons dry butter
  substitute
Vegetable cooking spray

STEPS IN PREPARATION:

1. Drain tomatoes, reserving liquid. Pour tomato liquid into a medium saucepan; bring to a boil. Add bouillon cube, stirring to dissolve.
2. Add tomato, bread, and next 3 ingredients. Sprinkle with butter substitute.
3. Transfer to a 1-quart casserole coated with cooking spray. Bake at 400° for 25 minutes or until thoroughly heated.

Yield: 8 servings

TURNIP GREENS

Exchanges: 2 Vegetable

Serving Size: ½ cup
Carbohydrate: 10 gm
Protein: 2 gm
Fat: 1 gm

Calories: 51
Fiber: 5 gm
Sodium: 273 mg
Cholesterol: 0 mg

INGREDIENTS:

2 pounds fresh turnip greens
3 cups water
½ teaspoon salt
½ cup chopped onion
2 teaspoons reduced-calorie margarine, melted

⅛ teaspoon ground allspice
1 tablespoon all-purpose flour
Sugar substitute to equal 1 teaspoon sugar*
2 tablespoons vinegar

STEPS IN PREPARATION:

1. Combine first 3 ingredients in large Dutch oven; bring to a boil. Reduce heat; simmer 1 hour or until tender.
2. Drain greens, reserving 1 cup liquid; set aside.
3. Sauté onion in margarine in a nonstick skillet. Add sautéed onion and allspice to drained greens.
4. Stir flour and sugar substitute into vinegar, stirring to dissolve; add to reserved 1 cup liquid. Add flour mixture to greens.
5. Cook over medium heat until thickened, stirring occasionally.

Yield: 6 servings

*See the sugar substitution chart on page 354.

MIXED VEGETABLE CASSEROLE

Exchanges: 2 Vegetable, ½ Fat

Serving Size: ½ cup	**Calories:** 66
Carbohydrate: 9 gm	**Fiber:** 2 gm
Protein: 3 gm	**Sodium:** 140 mg
Fat: 2 gm	**Cholesterol:** 4 mg

INGREDIENTS:

2 (10-ounce) packages frozen mixed vegetables

½ cup (2 ounces) shredded low-fat process American cheese

2 tablespoons chopped onion

2 tablespoons reduced-calorie mayonnaise

1 (8-ounce) can sliced water chestnuts, drained

Vegetable cooking spray

STEPS IN PREPARATION:

1. Cook mixed vegetables according to package directions, omitting salt and fat. Drain.
2. Combine mixed vegetables, cheese, and next 3 ingredients, stirring gently.
3. Spoon mixture into a 1½-quart casserole coated with cooking spray. Bake at 350° for 20 minutes or until thoroughly heated.

Yield: 8 servings

STIR-FRIED VEGETABLES

Exchanges: 1 Vegetable

Serving Size: 1 cup
Carbohydrate: 8 gm
Protein: 2 gm
Fat: trace

Calories: 41
Fiber: 1 gm
Sodium: 80 mg
Cholesterol: trace

INGREDIENTS:

Vegetable cooking spray
1 tablespoon reduced-sodium
  soy sauce
1 clove garlic, crushed
3 cups shredded cabbage
2 cups broccoli flowerets
1 cup sliced carrot
1 cup sliced green onions

2 cups sliced fresh
  mushrooms
1 (6-ounce) package frozen
  snow pea pods, thawed
1 cup water
1 tablespoon cornstarch
2 teaspoons chicken-flavored
  bouillon granules

STEPS IN PREPARATION:

1. Coat a wok or large nonstick skillet with cooking spray. Heat at medium-high (375°) until hot. Add soy sauce and garlic; stir-fry 3 minutes.
2. Add cabbage, broccoli, carrot, and green onions. Stir-fry 3 to 4 minutes or until vegetables are crisp-tender.
3. Add mushrooms and snow peas; stir-fry 2 minutes.
4. Combine water, cornstarch, and bouillon granules, stirring to dissolve. Pour over vegetable mixture, and stir-fry until thickened and bubbly.

Yield: 8 servings

MARINATED GARDEN VEGETABLES

Exchanges: 1 Vegetable, ½ Fat

Serving Size: ½ cup
Carbohydrate: 7 gm
Protein: 1 gm
Fat: 2 gm

Calories: 52
Fiber: 2 gm
Sodium: 310 mg
Cholesterol: 1 mg

INGREDIENTS:

2 cups broccoli flowerets
2 cups cauliflower flowerets
2 cups sliced carrot
½ cup chopped green pepper
½ cup sliced celery
1 medium zucchini, sliced

1 medium cucumber, sliced
Garden Vegetable Marinade
(page 295)
4 small tomatoes, cut into
quarters
1 cup sliced fresh mushrooms

STEPS IN PREPARATION:

1. Combine first 7 ingredients in a large bowl.
2. Pour Garden Vegetable Marinade over vegetables. Toss gently
   to coat.
3. Cover and marinate in refrigerator at least 12 hours, stirring occasionally. (Mixture can be stored in refrigerator up to 1 week.)
4. Add tomato and mushrooms just before serving.

Yield: 20 servings

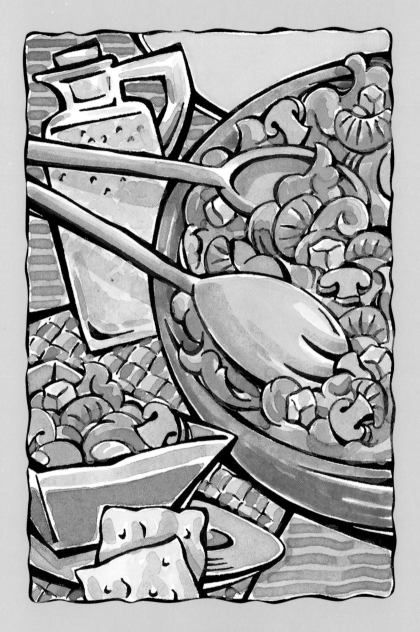

SALADS &
SALAD DRESSINGS

WALDORF SALAD

Exchanges: 1 Fruit, 1 Fat

Serving Size: ½ cup	**Calories:** 151
Carbohydrate: 10 gm	**Fiber:** 2 gm
Protein: trace	**Sodium:** 70 mg
Fat: 4 gm	**Cholesterol:** 0 mg

INGREDIENTS:

3 medium-size Red Delicious apples, cored and diced
½ cup sliced celery
¼ cup raisins

½ cup reduced-calorie mayonnaise
1 tablespoon lemon juice

STEPS IN PREPARATION:

1. Combine apple, celery, and raisins in a medium bowl.
2. Combine mayonnaise and lemon juice, stirring well. Add mayonaise mixture to fruit mixture, and toss lightly to coat.
3. Cover and chill.

Yield: 5 servings

Planning meals? Remember fruit salads are as satisfying as vegetable salads and can be used for any brunch, lunch, or dinner menu.

MIXED FRUIT SALAD

Exchanges: 1 Fruit

Serving Size: ⅓ cup
Carbohydrate: 15 gm
Protein: trace
Fat: trace

Calories: 57
Fiber: 1 gm
Sodium: 92 mg
Cholesterol: 0 mg

INGREDIENTS:

1 cup chopped apple
1 cup sliced banana
½ cup raisins
½ cup chopped celery
⅓ cup reduced-calorie
  mayonnaise

1 tablespoon lemon juice
1 (8-ounce) can pineapple
  chunks in juice, drained
Lettuce leaves (optional)

STEPS IN PREPARATION:

1. Combine first 7 ingredients in a medium bowl; toss gently to coat.
2. Cover and chill 1 hour.
3. Serve on lettuce leaves, if desired.

Yield: 16 servings

FRESH FRUIT SALAD

Exchanges: 1 Fruit

Serving Size: ½ cup
Carbohydrate: 9 gm
Protein: 1 gm
Fat: 1 gm

Calories: 47
Fiber: 1 gm
Sodium: 82 mg
Cholesterol: 0 mg

INGREDIENTS:

½ cup sliced fresh
  strawberries
½ cup seedless green grapes,
  cut in half
½ small cantaloupe, diced
¼ cup plain nonfat yogurt
2 tablespoons nonfat
  mayonnaise

1 tablespoon granulated
  brown sugar substitute
1 tablespoon chopped
  walnuts
Lettuce leaves (optional)

STEPS IN PREPARATION:

1. Combine strawberries, grapes, and cantaloupe.
2. Combine yogurt, mayonnaise, brown sugar substitute, and nuts,
   stirring well. Stir yogurt mixture into fruit mixture.
3. Serve on lettuce leaves, if desired.

Yield: 6 servings

SUMMER FRUIT SALAD IN LEMONADE GLAZE

Exchanges: 1 Fruit

Serving Size: 1 cup
Carbohydrate: 20 gm
Protein: 1 gm
Fat: 1 gm

Calories: 85
Fiber: 2 gm
Sodium: 3 mg
Cholesterol: 0 mg

INGREDIENTS:

1 (11-ounce) can mandarin oranges in water, undrained
¼ teaspoon unflavored gelatin
¼ cup frozen lemonade concentrate, thawed

1 teaspoon poppy seeds
2 cups fresh cherries, pitted and halved
2 cups sliced fresh peaches
1½ cups sliced fresh plums
Bibb lettuce leaves (optional)

STEPS IN PREPARATION:

1. Drain oranges, reserving ¼ cup liquid. Combine reserved liquid and gelatin in a small saucepan; let stand 1 minute. Stir in lemonade concentrate. Bring to a boil, and cook, stirring constantly, 2 minutes or until gelatin dissolves.
2. Remove from heat, and stir in poppy seeds. Cover and chill 3 hours or until thickened.
3. Combine oranges, cherries, peaches, and plums. Pour lemonade mixture over fruit mixture, and toss gently.

Yield: 6 servings

PINEAPPLE-ORANGE SALAD

Exchanges: 1 Fruit

Serving Size: ¼ cup	**Calories:** 64
Carbohydrate: 15 gm	**Fiber:** 1 gm
Protein: 2 gm	**Sodium:** 49 mg
Fat: trace	**Cholesterol:** 0 mg

INGREDIENTS:

2 envelopes unflavored gelatin

2 cups unsweetened orange juice, divided

2 cups canned crushed pineapple in juice, drained

Sugar substitute to equal ¼ cup sugar*

2 tablespoons lemon juice

½ teaspoon almond extract

¼ teaspoon salt

Vegetable cooking spray

STEPS IN PREPARATION:

1. Sprinkle gelatin over ½ cup orange juice to soften.
2. Heat remaining 1½ cups orange juice, and pour over softened gelatin mixture; stir until gelatin is dissolved.
3. Add pineapple and next 4 ingredients; stir well. Pour into a 3-cup mold coated with cooking spray; chill until set.
4. To serve, unmold onto a serving platter.

Yield: 12 servings

*See the sugar substitution chart on page 354.

PINEAPPLE-LIME SALAD

Exchanges: ½ Skim Milk

Serving Size: ½ cup
Carbohydrate: 5 gm
Protein: 5 gm
Fat: 1 gm

Calories: 50
Fiber: trace
Sodium: 112 mg
Cholesterol: 2 mg

INGREDIENTS:

1 (0.6-ounce) package sugar-free lime-flavored gelatin
2 cups boiling water
2 cups cold water
2 tablespoons reduced-calorie mayonnaise

1 cup 1% low-fat cottage cheese
1 (8¼-ounce) can crushed pineapple in juice, drained
Vegetable cooking spray
Lettuce leaves (optional)

STEPS IN PREPARATION:

1. Dissolve gelatin in boiling water in a medium bowl, stirring well. Stir in cold water. Chill until mixture is the consistency of unbeaten egg white.
2. Fold mayonnaise into gelatin mixture. Add cottage cheese and pineapple, stirring well.
3. Pour gelatin mixture into a 6-cup mold coated with cooking spray; chill gelatin mixture until set.
4. To serve, unmold onto lettuce leaves, if desired.

Yield: 10 servings

STRAWBERRY SALAD

Exchanges: 1 Fruit

Serving Size: ½ cup
Carbohydrate: 9 gm
Protein: 5 gm
Fat: trace

Calories: 60
Fiber: 1 gm
Sodium: 93 mg
Cholesterol: 1 mg

INGREDIENTS:

1 (3-ounce) package sugar-free strawberry gelatin
¾ cup chopped fresh strawberries
1 cup plain nonfat yogurt

Sugar substitute to equal 2 teaspoons sugar*
1 teaspoon vanilla extract
Vegetable cooking spray

STEPS IN PREPARATION:

1. Prepare gelatin according to package directions. Chill until slightly thickened.
2. Mash strawberries; add to gelatin mixture. Add yogurt, sugar substitute, and vanilla; stir until well blended.
3. Pour into 4 (½-cup) molds coated with cooking spray; chill until set.
4. To serve, unmold onto salad plates.

Yield: 4 servings

*See the sugar substitution chart on page 354.

CAESAR SALAD

Exchanges: ½ Starch, ½ Lean Meat, 1 Vegetable, ½ Fat

Serving Size: ¼ recipe
Carbohydrate: 13 gm
Protein: 5 gm
Fat: 4 gm

Calories: 114
Fiber: 1 gm
Sodium: 347 mg
Cholesterol: 3 mg

INGREDIENTS:

4 (½-inch-thick) slices French bread
Butter-flavored vegetable cooking spray
½ teaspoon garlic powder
6 cups torn romaine lettuce
2 tablespoons freshly grated Parmesan cheese
3½ tablespoons fresh lemon juice

1½ tablespoons water
1 tablespoon low-sodium Worcestershire sauce
2 teaspoons olive oil
¼ teaspoon garlic powder
6 anchovies, cut in half crosswise
Dash of freshly ground pepper

STEPS IN PREPARATION:

1. Cut bread into cubes; place on a baking sheet. Coat cubes with cooking spray; sprinkle with ½ teaspoon garlic powder. Broil 3 inches from heat (with electric oven door partially opened) until toasted on all sides, turning frequently.
2. Combine lettuce and cheese in a large bowl. Combine lemon juice and next 4 ingredients, stirring with a wire whisk until blended. Pour over lettuce mixture; toss gently.
3. Arrange lettuce mixture on salad plates, and top with anchovy halves. Sprinkle with bread cubes and freshly ground pepper. Serve immediately.

Yield: 4 servings

PICKLED BEET SALAD

Exchanges: 1 Vegetable

Serving Size: ½ cup	**Calories:** 35
Carbohydrate: 9 gm	**Fiber:** 2 gm
Protein: 1 gm	**Sodium:** 256 mg
Fat: trace	**Cholesterol:** 0 mg

INGREDIENTS:

3 cups canned beets in juice
¼ cup vinegar
Sugar substitute to equal 2
   tablespoons sugar*

½ teaspoon salt
¼ teaspoon ground cinnamon
⅛ teaspoon ground cloves
Dash of pepper

STEPS IN PREPARATION:

1. Drain beets, and place in a medium bowl; reserve juice in a saucepan.
2. Add vinegar and remaining ingredients to beet juice. Bring juice mixture to a boil; immediately remove from heat.
3. Pour juice mixture over beets.
4. Cover and chill; drain beets before serving.

Yield: 6 servings

*See the sugar substitution chart on page 354.

GREEN BEAN SALAD

Exchanges: 1 Vegetable, 1 Fat

Serving Size: ½ cup
Carbohydrate: 9 gm
Protein: 1 gm
Fat: 6 gm

Calories: 89
Fiber: 5 gm
Sodium: 880 mg
Cholesterol: 4 mg

INGREDIENTS:

2 (10-ounce) cans cut green
  beans, undrained
1 cup commercial no-oil
  Italian dressing
½ cup chopped dill pickles
½ teaspoon dried basil
½ teaspoon dried oregano
1 small red onion, sliced
1 clove garlic, minced

STEPS IN PREPARATION:

1. Place beans in a medium saucepan; cook over medium heat 5 minutes or until thoroughly heated. Drain.
2. Combine beans, Italian dressing, and remaining ingredients in a medium bowl; toss lightly to coat.
3. Cover and chill at least 8 hours.
4. Serve with a slotted spoon.

Yield: 4 servings

If you want to reduce sodium, use canned no-salt-added cut green beans in this recipe and others.

CARROT-RAISIN SALAD

Exchanges: 1 Fruit, 1 Vegetable

Serving Size: ¼ cup
Carbohydrate: 20 gm
Protein: 3 gm
Fat: trace

Calories: 86
Fiber: 2 gm
Sodium: 39 mg
Cholesterol: 1 mg

INGREDIENTS:

2 cups shredded carrot
1 cup canned crushed
   pineapple in juice, drained
½ cup raisins

1 (8-ounce) carton plain
   nonfat yogurt
Lettuce leaves (optional)

STEPS IN PREPARATION:

1. Combine carrot, pineapple, and raisins; stir well.
2. Cover and chill at least 2 hours.
3. Stir in yogurt, and serve on lettuce leaves, if desired.

Yield: 12 servings

CHILLED CAULIFLOWER SALAD

Exchanges: 1 Vegetable

Serving Size: ½ cup
Carbohydrate: 4 gm
Protein: 1 gm
Fat: 1 gm

Calories: 29
Fiber: 1 gm
Sodium: 170 mg
Cholesterol: 1 mg

INGREDIENTS:

1 medium cauliflower, broken into flowerets
½ cup sliced celery
½ cup commercial no-oil Italian dressing
¼ teaspoon salt
¼ teaspoon black pepper
¼ teaspoon ground red pepper
2 small cloves garlic, minced

STEPS IN PREPARATION:

1. Place cauliflower and water to cover in a medium saucepan; cover and bring to a boil. Cook 4 to 5 minutes or until crisp-tender. Drain.
2. Combine cooked cauliflower and celery in a medium bowl.
3. Combine Italian dressing and remaining ingredients, stirring well. Pour dressing mixture over cauliflower mixture, tossing gently to coat.
4. Cover and chill at least 2 hours.

Yield: 10 servings

MARINATED CUCUMBER SALAD

Exchanges: 1 Vegetable

Serving Size: ½ cup
Carbohydrate: 3 gm
Protein: trace
Fat: 2 gm

Calories: 35
Fiber: 1 gm
Sodium: 192 mg
Cholesterol: 1 mg

INGREDIENTS:

½ cup commercial no-oil Italian dressing
⅛ teaspoon pepper
1 medium cucumber, peeled and thinly sliced

½ small onion, thinly sliced
¼ cup thinly sliced radishes
2 tablespoons chopped fresh parsley

STEPS IN PREPARATION:

1. Combine Italian dressing and pepper in a medium bowl, stirring well. Add cucumber, onion, radishes, and parsley. Toss gently to coat.
2. Cover and marinate in refrigerator at least 4 hours.
3. Serve with a slotted spoon.

Yield: 5 servings

Add marinated vegetable salads to your next dinner party menu. They can be prepared in advance and chilled until serving time—an important time-saver for busy cooks.

COLESLAW

Exchanges: 1 Vegetable

Serving Size: ½ cup
Carbohydrate: 5 gm
Protein: 1 gm
Fat: trace

Calories: 23
Fiber: 1 gm
Sodium: 316 mg
Cholesterol: 0 mg

INGREDIENTS:

4 cups shredded cabbage
½ cup shredded carrot
⅓ cup nonfat mayonnaise
2 tablespoons prepared
   mustard

2 tablespoons vinegar
½ teaspoon salt

STEPS IN PREPARATION:

1. Combine all ingredients in a medium bowl. Toss gently to coat.
2. Cover and chill.

Yield: 8 servings

Select cabbage with fresh, crisp leaves that are firmly packed and a head that is heavy for its size. Cabbage will keep in the refrigerator, tightly wrapped in heavy-duty plastic wrap, for about two weeks.

CALIFORNIA COLESLAW

Exchanges: 1 Vegetable

Serving Size: ½ cup
Carbohydrate: 4 gm
Protein: trace
Fat: 1 gm

Calories: 22
Fiber: 1 gm
Sodium: 103 mg
Cholesterol: trace

INGREDIENTS:

1 cup shredded cabbage
1 cup shredded red cabbage
½ cup shredded carrot
½ cup chopped green pepper
½ cup chopped sweet red pepper
¼ cup chopped onion
1½ tablespoons minced fresh parsley

¼ cup vinegar
¼ cup commercial no-oil Italian dressing
Liquid sugar substitute to equal ¼ cup sugar*
⅛ teaspoon salt
⅛ teaspoon pepper

STEPS IN PREPARATION:

1. Combine first 7 ingredients in a large bowl, stirring well. Set aside.
2. Combine vinegar and remaining ingredients in a jar; cover tightly, and shake vigorously.
3. Pour dressing mixture over vegetables, tossing gently to coat.
4. Cover and chill.
5. To serve, stir coleslaw lightly, and serve with a slotted spoon.

Yield: 8 servings

*See the sugar substitution chart on page 354.

MARINATED COLESLAW

Exchanges: 1 Vegetable, ½ Fat

Serving Size: ½ cup
Carbohydrate: 7 gm
Protein: 1 gm
Fat: 3 gm

Calories: 59
Fiber: 2 gm
Sodium: 241 mg
Cholesterol: 2 mg

INGREDIENTS:

3 cups shredded cabbage
Sugar substitute to equal ¾
   cup sugar*
1 large green pepper, diced
1 large onion, diced

1½ cups commercial no-oil
    Italian dressing
1 tablespoon celery seeds
1 tablespoon dry mustard

STEPS IN PREPARATION:

1. Combine first 4 ingredients in a large bowl; stir well.
2. Combine Italian dressing, celery seeds, and dry mustard in a small saucepan. Bring to a boil, and remove from heat.
3. Pour dressing mixture over vegetable mixture, tossing gently to coat.
4. Cover and chill at least 1 hour.
5. To serve, stir coleslaw lightly, and serve with a slotted spoon.

Yield: 12 servings

*See the sugar substitution chart on page 354.

MARINATED VEGETABLE SALAD

Exchanges: 1 Vegetable

Serving Size: ½ cup
Carbohydrate: 11 gm
Protein: 1 gm
Fat: 1 gm

Calories: 56
Fiber: 2 gm
Sodium: 119 mg
Cholesterol: 1 mg

INGREDIENTS:

3 cups diagonally sliced
   carrot
1 cup chopped celery
½ cup chopped green pepper
1 teaspoon celery seeds
1 medium onion, thinly sliced

Sugar substitute to equal 1
   cup sugar*
½ cup commercial no-oil
   Italian salad dressing
¼ cup vinegar
¼ cup water

STEPS IN PREPARATION:

1. Place carrot in a small saucepan; cover with water, and boil 10 minutes or until crisp-tender. Drain well.
2. Place carrot, celery, and next 3 ingredients in a large shallow dish; toss lightly, and set aside.
3. Combine sugar substitute and remaining ingredients in a small saucepan, stirring well; bring to a boil, stirring frequently. Pour mixture over vegetables.
4. Cover and chill at least 8 hours.

Yield: 10 servings

*See the sugar substitution chart on page 354.

MACARONI SALAD

Exchanges: 1½ Starch, ½ Fat

Serving Size: ½ cup
Carbohydrate: 21 gm
Protein: 5 gm
Fat: 3 gm

Calories: 133
Fiber: 1 gm
Sodium: 366 mg
Cholesterol: 48 mg

INGREDIENTS:

1½ cups elbow macaroni, uncooked
¼ cup chopped green onions
2 hard-cooked eggs, chopped
2 dill pickles, chopped
½ cup commercial no-oil Italian dressing
2 tablespoons dill pickle juice
1 tablespoon prepared mustard
1 teaspoon dried dillweed

STEPS IN PREPARATION:

1. Cook macaroni according to package directions, omitting salt and fat. Drain well. Combine macaroni, onions, eggs, and chopped pickle in a large bowl.
2. Combine Italian dressing and remaining ingredients, stirring to blend. Pour over macaroni mixture; stir well to coat.
3. Cover and chill at least 1 hour.

Yield: 8 servings

POTATO SALAD

Exchanges: 1 Starch, ½ Medium-Fat Meat

Serving Size: ½ cup	**Calories:** 99
Carbohydrate: 15 gm	**Fiber:** 1 gm
Protein: 4 gm	**Sodium:** 243 mg
Fat: 3 gm	**Cholesterol:** 94 mg

INGREDIENTS:

2 medium baking potatoes
2 tablespoons diced celery
2 tablespoons prepared mustard
2 tablespoons reduced-calorie mayonnaise
2 teaspoons chopped onion
2 teaspoons chopped green pepper
2 teaspoons diced pimiento
2 teaspoons chopped dill pickle
2 hard-cooked eggs, chopped

STEPS IN PREPARATION:

1. Cook potatoes in boiling water to cover 30 minutes or until tender. Drain and cool slightly. Peel and dice potatoes.
2. Combine potato, celery, and remaining ingredients in a medium bowl, tossing to coat.
3. Cover and chill at least 1 hour.

Yield: 4 servings

TARRAGON POTATO SALAD

Exchanges: 1 Starch

Serving Size: ½ cup
Carbohydrate: 16 gm
Protein: 2 gm
Fat: 1 gm

Calories: 84
Fiber: 2 gm
Sodium: 124 mg
Cholesterol: 1 mg

INGREDIENTS:

1⅓ pounds round red
   potatoes, unpeeled
¾ teaspoon dried tarragon
½ teaspoon dried parsley
   flakes
½ teaspoon dry mustard

1 small clove garlic
½ cup commercial no-oil
   Italian dressing
¾ teaspoon lemon juice
2 tablespoons minced green
   onions

STEPS IN PREPARATION:

1. Cook potatoes in boiling water to cover 15 minutes or until tender.
   Drain well, and cool. Cut into ¼-inch slices, and set aside.
2. Combine tarragon, parsley, mustard, and garlic in container of an
   electric blender. Cover and process 30 seconds or until pureed.
   Add Italian dressing, and process until blended. With blender run-
   ning, slowly add lemon juice, and continue to process dressing
   mixture until smooth.
3. Add dressing mixture to cooked potato slices; add minced green
   onions, and toss well to coat.
4. Cover and chill.

Yield: 8 servings

TOMATO ASPIC

Exchanges: 1 Vegetable

Serving Size: ½ cup
Carbohydrate: 7 gm
Protein: 3 gm
Fat: trace

Calories: 35
Fiber: 1 gm
Sodium: 776 mg
Cholesterol: 0 mg

INGREDIENTS:

3 cups tomato juice
1 teaspoon salt
⅛ teaspoon pepper
2 lemon slices
1 stalk celery, sliced
1 small onion, sliced
1 bay leaf

⅔ cup chilled tomato juice
¼ cup vinegar
2 envelopes unflavored gelatin
¼ cup finely chopped celery
Vegetable cooking spray
Lettuce leaves (optional)

STEPS IN PREPARATION:

1. Combine first 7 ingredients in a medium saucepan. Simmer, uncovered, for 10 minutes. Strain mixture; remove and discard lemon slices, celery, onion, and bay leaf. Set aside, and keep warm.
2. Combine ⅔ cup tomato juice and vinegar; sprinkle gelatin over mixture to soften. Add warm juice mixture, stirring until gelatin dissolves.
3. Cover and chill until mixture begins to thicken.
4. Stir in chopped celery. Pour mixture into 7 (½-cup) molds coated with cooking spray; chill until set.
5. To serve, unmold on lettuce leaves, if desired.

Yield: 7 servings

SPINACH-MANDARIN SALAD

Exchanges: 1 Lean Meat, 1 Vegetable

Serving Size: 1 cup
Carbohydrate: 6 gm
Protein: 9 gm
Fat: 3 gm

Calories: 87
Fiber: 2 gm
Sodium: 317 mg
Cholesterol: 17 mg

INGREDIENTS:

4 cups fresh spinach
2 cups cherry tomatoes
1½ cups chopped cooked
   chicken breast (skinned
   before cooking and cooked
   without salt), chilled
1 cup thinly sliced radishes

½ pound fresh mushrooms,
   sliced
½ cup commercial croutons
   Mandarin Dressing (page 282)
2 tablespoons sesame seeds,
   toasted

STEPS IN PREPARATION:

1. Wash spinach leaves thoroughly in cold water; drain. Remove and discard stems.
2. Place spinach in a large bowl. Add tomatoes and next 4 ingredients.
3. Add Mandarin Dressing, and toss gently. Top with sesame seeds.

Yield: 10 servings

CHEF'S SALAD

Exchanges: 1 Lean Meat, 1 Vegetable

Serving Size: 1½ cups
Carbohydrate: 5 gm
Protein: 8 gm
Fat: 4 gm

Calories: 81
Fiber: 1 gm
Sodium: 262 mg
Cholesterol: 38 mg

INGREDIENTS:

8 cups torn iceberg lettuce
1 cup thinly sliced radishes
2 green onions, sliced
⅓ cup Thousand Island Dressing (page 283)
2 ounces chopped lean cooked ham
2 ounces chopped cooked turkey breast

2 (1-ounce) slices low-fat process American cheese, diced
1 (1-ounce) slice low-fat Swiss cheese, diced
2 small tomatoes, chopped
1 hard-cooked egg, chopped

STEPS IN PREPARATION:

1. Combine first 3 ingredients in a large bowl. Cover and chill.
2. Pour Thousand Island Dressing over vegetable mixture; toss gently to coat. Top with ham and remaining ingredients.

Yield: 8 servings

TURKEY SALAD

Exchanges: 1 Lean Meat, 1 Vegetable

Serving Size: 1 cup
Carbohydrate: 5 gm
Protein: 10 gm
Fat: 4 gm

Calories: 97
Fiber: 2 gm
Sodium: 487 mg
Cholesterol: 77 mg

INGREDIENTS:

2 cups chopped fresh spinach
5 ounces cooked turkey, cut into ½-inch strips
1 (10½-ounce) can asparagus spears, drained and chopped
2 medium tomatoes, sliced

2 hard-cooked eggs, chopped
1 green onion, chopped
¼ cup plus 2 tablespoons commercial no-oil Italian dressing
¼ cup prepared mustard

STEPS IN PREPARATION:

1. Combine first 6 ingredients in a large bowl. Cover and chill.
2. Combine Italian dressing and mustard, stirring until blended. Pour over salad, and toss gently to coat.
3. Cover and chill.

Yield: 6 servings

You don't have to cook an entire bird to enjoy the flavor of turkey. Check your local supermarket for small cuts such as turkey breast slices, tenderloins, or boneless turkey breast roasts.

CUCUMBER DRESSING

Exchanges: Free

Serving Size: 2 tablespoons
Carbohydrate: 2 gm
Protein: 1 gm
Fat: trace

Calories: 18
Fiber: trace
Sodium: 156 mg
Cholesterol: trace

INGREDIENTS:

1 small cucumber, peeled
½ teaspoon salt
½ cup plain low-fat yogurt
1 tablespoon reduced-calorie mayonnaise

¼ teaspoon lemon juice
1 tablespoon chopped fresh parsley
1 green onion, chopped
¼ teaspoon dried dillweed

STEPS IN PREPARATION:

1. Shred cucumber; spread on a paper towel. Sprinkle with salt. Let stand at room temperature 30 minutes. Squeeze excess moisture from cucumber.
2. Combine yogurt, mayonnaise, and lemon juice in a small bowl, stirring to blend. Stir in drained cucumber, parsley, green onion, and dillweed.
3. Cover and chill. Stir well before using.
4. Serve with salad greens.

Yield: 1 cup

Note: See the Vegetable List on page 22 for exchange values of salad greens.

FRENCH DRESSING

Exchanges: 1 Fat

Serving Size: 2 tablespoons
Carbohydrate: 3 gm
Protein: trace
Fat: 5 gm

Calories: 60
Fiber: trace
Sodium: 201 mg
Cholesterol: 0 mg

INGREDIENTS:

3 tablespoons vegetable oil
¾ teaspoon salt
½ teaspoon dry mustard
¼ teaspoon hot sauce

⅛ teaspoon paprika
1 cup unsweetened grapefruit
   juice, divided
2 teaspoons cornstarch

STEPS IN PREPARATION:

1. Combine first 5 ingredients in a small bowl, stirring well to blend. Set aside.
2. Combine ½ cup grapefruit juice and cornstarch in a small saucepan, stirring until blended. Cook over medium heat, stirring constantly, until mixture is thickened and bubbly. Remove from heat.
3. Add cornstarch mixture to oil mixture in bowl, and beat at medium speed of an electric mixer until smooth. Add remaining ½ cup grapefruit juice, and beat until dressing mixture is well blended.
4. Cover and chill.
5. Serve with salad greens.

Yield: 1 cup

Note: See the Vegetable List on page 22 for exchange values of salad greens.

HERB DRESSING
Exchanges: Free

Serving Size: 2 tablespoons
Carbohydrate: 2 gm
Protein: trace
Fat: 0 gm

Calories: 12
Fiber: 0 gm
Sodium: 0 mg
Cholesterol: 0 mg

INGREDIENTS:

½ cup white wine vinegar
¼ cup salad vinegar
1 teaspoon onion powder

1 teaspoon dried salad herbs
1 teaspoon lemon juice
½ teaspoon garlic powder

STEPS IN PREPARATION:

1. Combine all ingredients in a jar; cover tightly, and shake vigorously. Chill.
2. Shake well before using.
3. Serve with salad greens.

Yield: ¾ cup

Note: See the Vegetable List on page 22 for exchange values of salad greens.

ITALIAN DRESSING

Exchanges: 1 Fat

Serving Size: 2 tablespoons
Carbohydrate: 1 gm
Protein: trace
Fat: 5 gm

Calories: 49
Fiber: trace
Sodium: 111 mg
Cholesterol: 1 mg

INGREDIENTS:

¼ cup plus 2 tablespoons water
¼ cup vinegar
2 tablespoons chopped fresh parsley
2 tablespoons vegetable oil
1 tablespoon plus 1 teaspoon grated Parmesan cheese

2 teaspoons dry pectin
¼ teaspoon salt
¼ teaspoon pepper
¼ teaspoon dried Italian seasoning
1 large clove garlic, peeled

STEPS IN PREPARATION:

1. Combine first 9 ingredients in a jar; cover tightly, and shake vigorously.
2. Press a wooden pick through garlic clove; add garlic clove to dressing mixture. Cover and chill.
3. To serve, remove and discard garlic. Cover and shake well before using.
4. Serve with salad greens.

Yield: ¾ cup

Note: See the Vegetable List on page 22 for exchange values of salad greens.

MANDARIN DRESSING
Exchanges: ½ Fat

Serving Size: 2 tablespoons
Carbohydrate: 4 gm
Protein: 1 gm
Fat: 3 gm

Calories: 42
Fiber: 1 gm
Sodium: 558 mg
Cholesterol: 1 mg

INGREDIENTS:

¼ cup commercial no-oil
  Italian dressing
Sugar substitute to equal 2
  tablespoons sugar*
2 tablespoons reduced-sodium
  soy sauce

1 teaspoon vinegar
1 teaspoon sesame seeds
⅛ teaspoon pepper

STEPS IN PREPARATION:

1. Combine all ingredients in a jar; cover tightly, and shake vigorously.
2. Chill at least 2 hours to blend flavors.
3. Serve over vegetable salads.

Yield: ¼ cup plus 2 tablespoons

Note: See the Vegetable List on page 22 for exchange values of vegetables.

*See the sugar substitution chart on page 354.

THOUSAND ISLAND DRESSING

Exchanges: Free

Serving Size: 2 tablespoons	**Calories:** 21
Carbohydrate: 2 gm	**Fiber:** trace
Protein: 1 gm	**Sodium:** 109 mg
Fat: 1 gm	**Cholesterol:** trace

INGREDIENTS:

¼ cup plain low-fat yogurt
¼ cup nonfat buttermilk
1 tablespoon reduced-calorie mayonnaise
1 tablespoon chopped dill pickle
1 tablespoon reduced-calorie ketchup
1 teaspoon chopped fresh parsley
⅛ teaspoon salt

STEPS IN PREPARATION:

1. Combine yogurt, buttermilk, and mayonnaise in a small bowl, stirring until blended. Stir in pickle and remaining ingredients.
2. Cover and chill.
3. Serve with salad greens.

Yield: ¾ cup

Note: See the Vegetable List on page 22 for exchange values of salad greens.

VINEGAR SALAD DRESSING

Exchanges: Free

Serving Size: 2 tablespoons
Carbohydrate: 4 gm
Protein: trace
Fat: trace

Calories: 15
Fiber: 0 gm
Sodium: 135 mg
Cholesterol: 0 mg

INGREDIENTS:

1 cup apple vinegar
2 tablespoons lemon juice
Sugar substitute to equal 4
  teaspoons sugar*
2 teaspoons finely chopped
  onion

1 teaspoon paprika
½ teaspoon salt
½ teaspoon dry mustard

STEPS IN PREPARATION:

1. Combine all ingredients in a jar; cover tightly, and shake vigorously. Chill.
2. Shake well before using.
3. Serve with salad greens.

Yield: 1 cup

Note: See the Vegetable List on page 22 for exchange values of salad greens.

*See the sugar substitution chart on page 354.

YOGURT-FRUIT SALAD DRESSING

Exchanges: Free

Serving Size: 2 tablespoons
Carbohydrate: 3 gm
Protein: 1 gm
Fat: trace

Calories: 17
Fiber: trace
Sodium: 233 mg
Cholesterol: trace

INGREDIENTS:

1 teaspoon grated orange rind
2 tablespoons unsweetened
orange juice
2 tablespoons lemon juice

1 teaspoon salt
½ teaspoon dry mustard
¼ teaspoon paprika
1 cup plain low-fat yogurt

STEPS IN PREPARATION:

1. Combine first 6 ingredients in a small bowl, stirring until well blended; gently fold in yogurt.
2. Cover and chill.
3. Serve with fresh fruit salad.

Yield: 1¼ cups

Note: See the Fruit List on page 23 for exchange values of fruit.

ZERO SALAD DRESSING
Exchanges: Free

Serving Size: 2 tablespoons
Carbohydrate: 2 gm
Protein: trace
Fat: trace

Calories: 8
Fiber: 0 gm
Sodium: 178 mg
Cholesterol: 0 mg

INGREDIENTS:

½ cup tomato juice
2 tablespoons lemon juice or vinegar
1 tablespoon minced onion

⅛ teaspoon salt
⅛ teaspoon dried oregano
Dash of garlic powder
Dash of pepper

STEPS IN PREPARATION:

1. Combine all ingredients in a jar; cover tightly, and shake vigorously. Chill.
2. Shake well before using.
3. Serve with salad greens.

Yield: ½ cup

Note: See the Vegetable List on page 22 for exchange values of salad greens.

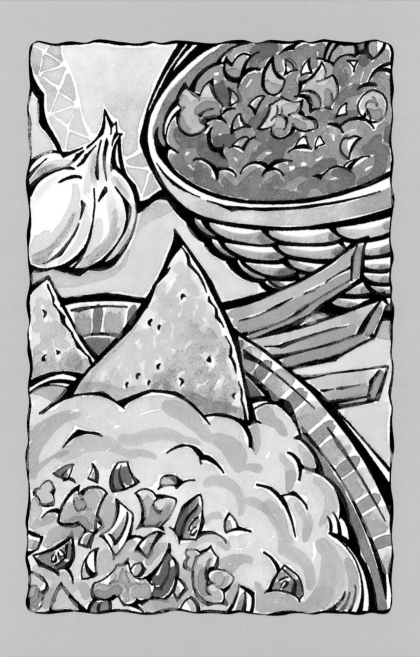

SAUCES & TOPPINGS

HORSERADISH SAUCE

Exchanges: Free

Serving Size: 1 tablespoon	**Calories:** 11
Carbohydrate: 2 gm	**Fiber:** trace
Protein: 1 gm	**Sodium:** 28 mg
Fat: trace	**Cholesterol:** 0 mg

INGREDIENTS:

1 (8-ounce) carton nonfat
  sour cream
¼ cup minced fresh parsley
¼ cup prepared horseradish

1 teaspoon white wine
  Worcestershire sauce
⅛ teaspoon pepper

STEPS IN PREPARATION:

1. Combine sour cream, parsley, horseradish, Worcestershire sauce, and pepper in a small bowl, stirring well to combine. Cover and chill.
2. Serve with beef or pork.

Yield: 1 cup

Note: See the Meat List on page 19 for exchange values of meat and poultry.

ZESTY BARBECUE SAUCE

Exchanges: Free

Serving Size: 2 tablespoons
Carbohydrate: 3 gm
Protein: trace
Fat: trace

Calories: 13
Fiber: 0 gm
Sodium: 135 mg
Cholesterol: 0 mg

INGREDIENTS:

½ cup lemon juice
⅓ cup cider vinegar
¼ cup cold water
¼ cup tomato juice
Sugar substitute to equal 4
  teaspoons sugar*
1 teaspoon dry mustard
1 teaspoon hot sauce

½ teaspoon salt
½ teaspoon onion powder
½ teaspoon paprika
½ teaspoon ground red
  pepper
½ teaspoon black pepper
⅛ teaspoon garlic powder
⅛ teaspoon dried oregano

STEPS IN PREPARATION:

1. Combine all ingredients in a medium saucepan. Bring mixture to a boil.
2. Transfer mixture to a serving container; cover and chill.
3. Serve with meat or poultry.

Yield: 1¼ cups

Note: See the Meat List on page 19 for exchange values of meat and poultry.

*See the sugar substitution chart on page 354.

CHEESE SAUCE

Exchanges: ½ Skim Milk, ½ Fat

Serving Size: ¼ cup	**Calories:** 78
Carbohydrate: 6 gm	**Fiber:** 0 gm
Protein: 6 gm	**Sodium:** 539 mg
Fat: 4 gm	**Cholesterol:** 9 mg

INGREDIENTS:

1 tablespoon all-purpose flour
1 cup skim milk, divided
1 tablespoon reduced-calorie margarine

½ cup (2 ounces) shredded low-fat process American cheese
½ teaspoon salt

STEPS IN PREPARATION:

1. Combine flour and ¼ cup milk; stir until smooth. Combine flour mixture, remaining ¾ cup milk, and margarine in a small saucepan; stir well. Cook over medium heat, stirring constantly, until mixture is thickened and bubbly.
2. Add shredded cheese and salt. Cook, stirring constantly, until cheese melts. (Do not overcook.)
3. Serve over vegetables.

Yield: 1 cup

Note: See the Vegetable List on page 22 for exchange values of vegetables.

COCKTAIL SAUCE
Exchanges: Free

Serving Size: 2 tablespoons
Carbohydrate: 4 gm
Protein: 1 gm
Fat: trace

Calories: 19
Fiber: 1 gm
Sodium: 459 mg
Cholesterol: 0 mg

INGREDIENTS:

½ cup tomato sauce
Sugar substitute to equal 2
   teaspoons sugar*
1 teaspoon finely chopped
   parsley
1 teaspoon lemon juice

½ teaspoon salt
½ teaspoon horseradish
½ teaspoon Worcestershire
   sauce
⅛ teaspoon dried oregano
Dash of onion powder

STEPS IN PREPARATION:

1. Combine all ingredients in a small bowl; stir well. Cover and chill.
2. Serve with baked, boiled, or broiled seafood.

Yield: ½ cup

Note: See the Meat List on page 19 for exchange values of seafood.

*See the sugar substitution chart on page 354.

FAT-FREE BEEF GRAVY

Exchanges: Free

Serving Size: 2 tablespoons
Carbohydrate: 1 gm
Protein: trace
Fat: 0 gm

Calories: 5
Fiber: 0 gm
Sodium: 76 mg
Cholesterol: 0 mg

INGREDIENTS:

2 tablespoons cornstarch or arrowroot
2 cups fat-free meat drippings or fat-free beef broth, divided
¼ teaspoon salt
¼ teaspoon pepper

½ cup minced onion (optional)
½ cup chopped mushrooms (optional)
2 tablespoons minced parsley (optional)

STEPS IN PREPARATION:

1. Add cornstarch to ½ cup broth, and stir.
2. Heat remaining 1½ cups broth in a saucepan. Add cornstarch mixture to hot broth. Add salt, pepper, and, if desired, onion, mushrooms, and parsley.
3. Reduce heat, and simmer, stirring constantly, until mixture thickens.

Yield: 3 cups

To make fat-free meat drippings, chill juices from cooked meats, and then skim off and discard fat. Use the fat-free juices for gravy or seasoning vegetables.

FAT-FREE CHICKEN GRAVY

Exchanges: Free

Serving Size: 2 tablespoons
Carbohydrate: 2 gm
Protein: 1 gm
Fat: trace

Calories: 15
Fiber: 0 gm
Sodium: 167 mg
Cholesterol: 0 mg

INGREDIENTS:

2 tablespoons all-purpose
  flour
¼ cup skim milk
1 cup fat-free chicken broth

½ teaspoon dried onion
  flakes
¼ teaspoon salt
¼ teaspoon pepper

STEPS IN PREPARATION:

1. Add flour to skim milk; stir until smooth.
2. Place broth and onion in a saucepan; bring to a boil.
3. Gradually add flour mixture to broth mixture, stirring constantly; stir in salt and pepper. Reduce heat; cook, stirring constantly, 5 minutes.

Yield: 1 cup

Cornstarch and flour are two of the most common thickening agents for sauces. Sauces that are thickened with flour look creamy; cornstarch-thickened sauces appear more transparent.

GUACAMOLE

Exchanges: 1 Fat

Serving Size: 2 tablespoons	**Calories:** 50
Carbohydrate: 3 gm	**Fiber:** 1 gm
Protein: trace	**Sodium:** 166 mg
Fat: 4 gm	**Cholesterol:** 0 mg

INGREDIENTS:

2 large avocados, peeled, seeded, and mashed

3 canned green chiles, seeded and chopped

3 tablespoons lemon or lime juice

¼ teaspoon salt

STEPS IN PREPARATION:

1. Combine avocado and green chiles in a medium bowl, stirring to blend.
2. Add lemon juice and salt, stirring well. Cover and chill.
3. Serve with tortilla chips or as a topping for meat or poultry.

Yield: 1½ cups

Note: See the Starch List on page 16 for exchange values of chips and the Meat List on page 19 for exchange values of meat and poultry.

Serve red or blue corn tortilla chips with Guacamole for a festive look. The chips are made from naturally pigmented red and blue corn kernals. Red or blue chips can be found in specialty supermarkets and health food stores. Be sure to look for the low-salt, low-fat varieties.

GARDEN VEGETABLE MARINADE

Exchanges: Free

Serving Size: 2 tablespoons
Carbohydrate: 3 gm
Protein: trace
Fat: trace

Calories: 12
Fiber: trace
Sodium: 161 mg
Cholesterol: 0 mg

INGREDIENTS:

2 cups commercial no-oil
  Italian dressing
Sugar substitute to equal ¾
  cup sugar*

1 teaspoon salt
2 cloves garlic, crushed

STEPS IN PREPARATION:

1. Combine all ingredients in a jar. Cover tightly, and shake vigorously. Store in refrigerator.
2. Use as a marinade for fresh vegetables.

Yield: 2 cups

Note: See the Vegetable List on page 22 for exchange values of vegetables.

*See the sugar substitution chart on page 354.

SALSA

Exchanges: Free

Serving Size: 2 tablespoons	**Calories:** 16
Carbohydrate: 2 gm	**Fiber:** trace
Protein: trace	**Sodium:** 313 mg
Fat: trace	**Cholesterol:** 0 mg

INGREDIENTS:

2 medium tomatoes, peeled and chopped
3 tablespoons canned diced green chiles, drained

2 tablespoons minced onion
1 teaspoon vegetable oil
1 teaspoon vinegar
½ teaspoon salt

STEPS IN PREPARATION:

1. Combine all ingredients in a medium bowl, stirring well.
2. Transfer mixture to a serving container; cover and chill.
3. Serve with tortilla chips or as a topping for meat or poultry.

Yield: 1 cup

Note: See the Starch List on page 16 for exchange values of chips and the Meat List on page 19 for exchange values of meat and poultry.

Enjoy the convenience of low-fat snack products now available such as no-oil baked tortilla chips, fat-free potato chips, fat-free crackers, and baked rice snacks.

MEATLESS TOMATO SAUCE

Exchanges: 1 Vegetable

Serving Size: ½ cup	**Calories:** 28
Carbohydrate: 6 gm	**Fiber:** 1 gm
Protein: 1 gm	**Sodium:** 452 mg
Fat: trace	**Cholesterol:** 0 mg

INGREDIENTS:

1 (16-ounce) can no-salt-added whole tomatoes, undrained and chopped
1 tablespoon dried basil
1 teaspoon garlic powder
½ teaspoon salt
⅛ teaspoon pepper

STEPS IN PREPARATION:

1. Combine all ingredients in a medium saucepan, stirring until well blended.
2. Bring tomato mixture to a boil; reduce heat, and simmer, uncovered, 30 minutes, stirring occasionally.
3. Serve over cooked noodles (cooked without salt or fat).

Yield: 2 cups

Note: See the Starch List on page 16 for exchange value of noodles.

WHITE SAUCE

Exchanges: Free

Serving Size: 2 tablespoons
Carbohydrate: 2 gm
Protein: 1 gm
Fat: 1 gm

Calories: 20
Fiber: 0 gm
Sodium: 166 mg
Cholesterol: 1 mg

INGREDIENTS:

1 tablespoon all-purpose
  flour
1 cup skim milk, divided

1 tablespoon reduced-calorie
  margarine
½ teaspoon salt

STEPS IN PREPARATION:

1. Combine flour and ¼ cup milk; stir until smooth. Combine flour
   mixture, remaining ¾ cup milk, and margarine in a small
   saucepan; stir well. Cook over medium heat, stirring constantly,
   until mixture is thickened and bubbly.
2. Remove from heat, and stir in salt.
3. Serve with fish, meat, or poultry.

Yield: 1 cup

Note: See the Meat List on page 19 for exchange values of fish,
meat, and poultry.

APPLE JELLY

Exchanges: Free

Serving Size: 1 tablespoon	**Calories:** 13
Carbohydrate: 3 gm	**Fiber:** 0 gm
Protein: trace	**Sodium:** 1 mg
Fat: trace	**Cholesterol:** 0 mg

INGREDIENTS:

1½ cups unsweetened apple juice
¾ teaspoon lemon juice
6 whole cloves
1 stick cinnamon

1½ teaspoons unflavored gelatin
⅓ cup cold water
Sugar substitute to equal ½ cup sugar*

STEPS IN PREPARATION:

1. Combine first 4 ingredients in a heavy saucepan. Bring to a boil; reduce heat, and simmer 10 minutes.
2. Sprinkle gelatin over cold water; let stand 1 minute.
3. Remove juice mixture from heat; remove and discard cloves and cinnamon. Add gelatin mixture and sugar substitute, stirring until gelatin dissolves.
4. Pour carefully into 2 hot (8-ounce) jars. Cover lightly until cooled. Cover tightly, and store in refrigerator.
5. Serve with bread, toast, or crackers.

Yield: 1⅓ cups

Note: See the Starch List on page 16 for exchange values of bread, toast, and crackers.

*See the sugar substitution chart on page 354.

CRANBERRY SAUCE

Exchanges: Free

Serving Size: 2 tablespoons
Carbohydrate: 8 gm
Protein: trace
Fat: trace

Calories: 32
Fiber: 0 gm
Sodium: 19 mg
Cholesterol: 0 mg

INGREDIENTS:

Sugar substitute to equal 1
  cup sugar*
½ cup water
2 tablespoons grated
  orange rind

¼ teaspoon salt
⅛ teaspoon ground cinnamon
Dash of cloves
4 cups fresh ripe cranberries
½ teaspoon vanilla extract

STEPS IN PREPARATION:

1. Combine first 6 ingredients in a medium saucepan. Bring to a boil; reduce heat, and simmer 5 minutes, stirring occasionally.
2. Add cranberries; simmer 10 to 15 minutes or until skins pop. Remove from heat, and add vanilla. Cover and chill.
3. Serve with baked chicken or turkey.

Yield: 3¾ cups

Note: See the Meat List on page 19 for exchange values of chicken and turkey.

*See the sugar substitution chart on page 354.

STRAWBERRY SAUCE

Exchanges: Free

Serving Size: 1 tablespoon	**Calories:** 11
Carbohydrate: 3 gm	**Fiber:** trace
Protein: trace	**Sodium:** 3 mg
Fat: trace	**Cholesterol:** 0 mg

INGREDIENTS:

1 quart fresh strawberries, washed, hulled, and coarsely chopped
¾ cup cold water, divided
2 tablespoons lemon juice

¼ teaspoon ground cinnamon
3 tablespoons cornstarch
Sugar substitute to equal 1 cup sugar*

STEPS IN PREPARATION:

1. Combine strawberries, ½ cup water, lemon juice, and cinnamon in a small Dutch oven, stirring well; bring mixture to a boil.
2. Dissolve cornstarch in remaining ¼ cup water, and stir into strawberry mixture. Reduce heat, and simmer 2 to 3 minutes or until mixture thickens, stirring occasionally.
3. Remove from heat, and let cool. Stir in sugar substitute.
4. Serve with pancakes, waffles, or toast.

Yield: 2 cups

Note: See the Starch List on page 16 for exchange values of pancakes, waffles, and toast.

*See the sugar substitution chart on page 354.

WHIPPED TOPPING

Exchanges: Free

Serving Size: ¼ cup
Carbohydrate: 2 gm
Protein: trace
Fat: trace

Calories: 10
Fiber: 0 gm
Sodium: 10 mg
Cholesterol: trace

INGREDIENTS:

¼ cup ice water
¼ cup instant nonfat dry
   milk powder

Sugar substitute to equal ⅓
   cup sugar*
1 tablespoon lemon juice

STEPS IN PREPARATION:

1. Place ice water in a small bowl; gradually add milk powder, beating at high speed of an electric mixer until stiff peaks form.
2. Gently fold in sugar substitute and lemon juice. Cover and chill.
3. Use as a substitute for whipped cream.

Yield: 2½ cups

*See the sugar substitution chart on page 354.

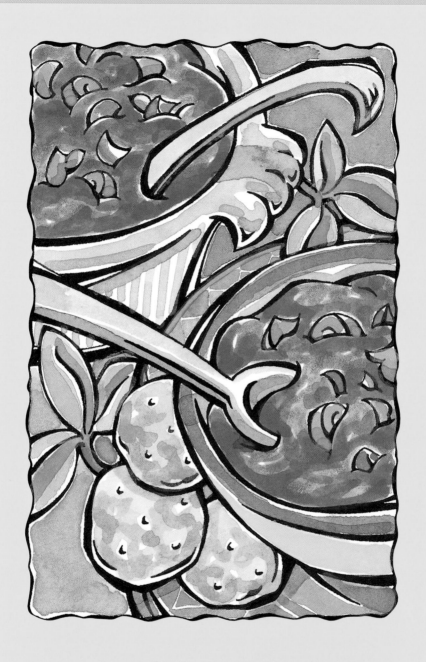

SOUPS

BROCCOLI-CAULIFLOWER SOUP

Exchanges: 1 Vegetable

Serving Size: ½ cup
Carbohydrate: 5 gm
Protein: 3 gm
Fat: trace

Calories: 32
Fiber: 1 gm
Sodium: 274 mg
Cholesterol: 1 mg

INGREDIENTS:

1½ cups water
1 (10-ounce) package frozen
　chopped broccoli, thawed
1 (10-ounce) package frozen
　cauliflower, thawed
⅓ cup chopped onion
2 teaspoons chicken-flavored
　bouillon granules

¼ teaspoon ground mace
1 tablespoon cornstarch
3 cups skim milk, divided
½ teaspoon salt
⅛ teaspoon pepper

STEPS IN PREPARATION:

1. Combine first 5 ingredients in a small Dutch oven. Cover and bring to a boil. Cook 5 to 8 minutes or until vegetables are tender (do not drain). Stir in mace.
2. Transfer vegetable mixture in batches to container of an electric blender or food processor; cover and process until smooth.
3. Return vegetable mixture to Dutch oven.
4. Dissolve cornstarch in ½ cup milk; stir into vegetable mixture.
5. Add remaining 2½ cups milk, salt, and pepper to vegetable mixture, stirring well.
6. Cook over medium heat until mixture is thickened and bubbly, stirring frequently.

Yield: 15 servings

FLAVORFUL ONION SOUP

Exchanges: 1 Vegetable

Serving Size: 2 cups	**Calories:** 24
Carbohydrate: 3 gm	**Fiber:** trace
Protein: trace	**Sodium:** 45 mg
Fat: 2 gm	**Cholesterol:** 0 mg

INGREDIENTS:

1 tablespoon reduced-calorie margarine
1 medium onion, thinly sliced
5½ cups water
1 tablespoon plus 2 teaspoons low-sodium beef-flavored bouillon granules

½ teaspoon Worcestershire sauce

STEPS IN PREPARATION:

1. Melt margarine in a medium saucepan over low heat; add onion. Cover and cook over low heat 20 minutes or until onion is lightly browned, stirring occasionally.
2. Add water, bouillon granules, and Worcestershire sauce, stirring well.
3. Cover and bring to a boil. Reduce heat, and simmer 10 minutes.

Yield: 3 servings

ENGLISH PEA SOUP

Exchanges: ½ Starch

Serving Size: ½ cup
Carbohydrate: 8 gm
Protein: 3 gm
Fat: trace

Calories: 45
Fiber: 3 gm
Sodium: 372 mg
Cholesterol: trace

INGREDIENTS:

1 (10-ounce) package frozen
   English peas
¼ medium head lettuce
3 ounces fresh spinach
½ cup chopped green onions
2 teaspoons chicken-flavored
   bouillon granules

½ teaspoon dried chervil,
   crushed
⅛ teaspoon pepper
1¼ cups water
¾ cup skim milk

STEPS IN PREPARATION:

1. Combine first 7 ingredients in a medium saucepan; stir in water.
   Cover and bring to a boil; reduce heat, and simmer 20 minutes.
2. Transfer mixture to container of an electric blender or food
   processor; cover and process until smooth.
3. Return mixture to saucepan; stir in milk.
4. Cook over medium heat until thoroughly heated, stirring frequently.

Yield: 8 servings

CREAMED POTATO SOUP

Exchanges: 1 Starch

Serving Size: ¾ cup
Carbohydrate: 14 gm
Protein: 2 gm
Fat: trace

Calories: 65
Fiber: 1 gm
Sodium: 144 mg
Cholesterol: trace

INGREDIENTS:

4 medium round red
  potatoes, peeled and sliced
1 small onion, peeled and
  sliced
4 green onions, coarsely
  chopped
2 (10½-ounce) cans no-salt-
  added chicken broth,
  undiluted

1 clove garlic, minced
1 cup skim milk
½ teaspoon salt
⅛ teaspoon ground white
  pepper
⅛ teaspoon ground nutmeg

STEPS IN PREPARATION:

1. Combine first 5 ingredients in a heavy 3-quart saucepan. Cover
   and simmer 20 minutes or until potato is tender.
2. Transfer potato mixture in batches to container of an electric
   blender or food processor; cover and process until smooth.
3. Combine pureed mixture with milk and remaining ingredients,
   stirring until well blended. Serve warm or chilled.

Yield: 9 servings

Reduce calories, fat, and cholesterol in cream-
based soups by using skim milk in place of
whipping cream or half-and-half.

TOMATO BOUILLON

Exchanges: 1 Vegetable

Serving Size: ¾ cup
Carbohydrate: 4 gm
Protein: 1 gm
Fat: trace

Calories: 17
Fiber: 1 gm
Sodium: 343 mg
Cholesterol: 0 mg

INGREDIENTS:

1¾ cups water
1½ cups tomato juice
2 teaspoons low-sodium
  beef-flavored bouillon
  granules

1 teaspoon Worcestershire
  sauce
⅛ teaspoon hot sauce

STEPS IN PREPARATION:

1. Combine all ingredients in a medium saucepan, stirring until bouillon granules dissolve.
2. Cover and bring to a boil. Reduce heat, and simmer 10 minutes.

Yield: 4 servings

No-salt-added tomato juice will make this recipe lower in sodium.

VEGETABLE-CHEESE SOUP

Exchanges: 1 Vegetable, ½ Skim Milk

Serving Size: 1 cup
Carbohydrate: 12 gm
Protein: 4 gm
Fat: 1 gm

Calories: 71
Fiber: 2 gm
Sodium: 384 mg
Cholesterol: 3 mg

INGREDIENTS:

1 (10-ounce) package frozen
  mixed vegetables, thawed
1 small onion, diced
2 tablespoons all-purpose
  flour
1 teaspoon dried Italian
  seasoning
¼ teaspoon salt
⅛ teaspoon pepper

1 cup water
1 cup skim milk
1 teaspoon chicken-flavored
  bouillon granules
¼ cup (1 ounce) shredded
  low-fat process American
  cheese
2 teaspoons Dijon mustard

STEPS IN PREPARATION:

1. Combine mixed vegetables and onion in a medium saucepan.
2. Combine flour, Italian seasoning, salt, and pepper, stirring well; add to vegetables, and stir to coat.
3. Combine water and milk; add bouillon granules, stirring until granules dissolve. Add to vegetable mixture, and bring to a boil.
4. Cook, stirring constantly, 5 minutes or until mixture is thickened and bubbly.
5. Reduce heat to low; add cheese and mustard, stirring to blend. Serve immediately.

Yield: 6 servings

ZUCCHINI SOUP

Exchanges: 1 Starch

Serving Size: 1 cup
Carbohydrate: 22 gm
Protein: 4 gm
Fat: 2 gm

Calories: 108
Fiber: 4 gm
Sodium: 65 mg
Cholesterol: trace

INGREDIENTS:

5 cups chopped zucchini
1 large baking potato, peeled and cut into 1-inch cubes
1 cup water
3 green onions, thinly sliced
1 tablespoon reduced-calorie margarine, melted

½ cup water
1½ teaspoons dried tarragon
½ teaspoon chicken-flavored bouillon granules
½ cup skim milk

STEPS IN PREPARATION:

1. Combine zucchini, potato, and 1 cup water in a small Dutch oven. Cover and bring to a boil. Boil 10 minutes or until crisp-tender (do not drain).
2. Sauté onions in margarine in a nonstick skillet until tender; add to zucchini mixture. Add ½ cup water, tarragon, and bouillon granules, stirring to blend.
3. Add skim milk, and cook over medium heat until thoroughly heated, stirring frequently.

Yield: 4 servings

QUICK BEEF SOUP

Exchanges: 1 Medium-Fat Meat, 1½ Vegetable

Serving Size: ½ cup
Carbohydrate: 9 gm
Protein: 7 gm
Fat: 4 gm

Calories: 98
Fiber: 2 gm
Sodium: 420 mg
Cholesterol: 16 mg

INGREDIENTS:

½ pound ground chuck
2 cups sliced carrot
¼ cup chopped onion
2 (8-ounce) cans tomato
   sauce

1 (2½-ounce) jar sliced
   mushrooms, drained
2 cups water

STEPS IN PREPARATION:

1. Cook ground chuck in a large nonstick skillet over medium heat until browned, stirring until meat crumbles. Drain and pat dry with paper towels. Wipe pan drippings from skillet with a paper towel.
2. Return meat to skillet; add carrot, onion, tomato sauce, and mushrooms. Stir in water.
3. Cover and bring to a boil. Reduce heat, and simmer 30 to 35 minutes or until carrot is tender, stirring occasionally.

Yield: 8 servings

GARDEN CHICKEN SOUP

Exchanges: 1 Starch, ½ Lean Meat

Serving Size: 1 cup
Carbohydrate: 16 gm
Protein: 6 gm
Fat: 1 gm

Calories: 101
Fiber: 2 gm
Sodium: 267 mg
Cholesterol: 8 mg

INGREDIENTS:

6 cups water
2 cups tomato juice
1 cup peeled, diced potato
1 cup chopped onion
1 cup whole kernel corn
1 cup cooked, drained lima beans
¾ cup chopped cooked chicken breast (skinned before cooking and cooked without salt)

½ cup sliced carrot
½ cup chopped celery
2 tablespoons low-sodium chicken-flavored bouillon granules
1 teaspoon garlic powder
1½ teaspoons Worcestershire sauce

STEPS IN PREPARATION:

1. Combine all ingredients in a large Dutch oven. Cover and bring to a boil.
2. Reduce heat, and simmer 45 minutes.

Yield: 10 servings

Simple garnishes such as a sprinkling of fresh herbs or green onions, a slice of lemon, or a teaspoon of nonfat sour cream give soups an added touch of flavor and color.

NAVY BEAN SOUP
Exchanges: 2 Starch

Serving Size: 1 cup
Carbohydrate: 30 gm
Protein: 9 gm
Fat: 1 gm

Calories: 160
Fiber: 8 gm
Sodium: 283 mg
Cholesterol: 0 mg

INGREDIENTS:

1 (16-ounce) package dried
   navy beans
2 quarts water
1½ cups diced onion
¼ cup diced celery

1 tablespoon reduced-calorie
   margarine, melted
2 cups canned stewed
   tomatoes, drained
1 teaspoon salt

STEPS IN PREPARATION:

1. Sort and wash beans; place in a large Dutch oven. Cover with water 2 inches above beans; soak overnight. Drain beans.
2. Combine beans and 2 quarts water; bring to a boil. Cover, reduce heat, and simmer 2 hours.
3. Sauté onion and celery in margarine until tender; add onion mixture, tomato, and salt to bean mixture, stirring well.
4. Simmer, uncovered, 1 hour or until beans are tender.

Yield: 11 servings

COUNTRY CHILI

Exchanges: 1 Starch

Serving Size: ⅔ cup
Carbohydrate: 15 gm
Protein: 4 gm
Fat: 1 gm

Calories: 85
Fiber: 4 gm
Sodium: 598 mg
Cholesterol: 0 mg

INGREDIENTS:

1 large onion, chopped
1 clove garlic, chopped
1 tablespoon reduced-calorie margarine, melted
1 teaspoon salt
1 teaspoon dried basil
1 teaspoon chili powder
½ teaspoon dried oregano

½ teaspoon dried thyme
¼ teaspoon pepper
1 (16-ounce) can whole tomatoes, undrained and chopped
1 (8-ounce) can red kidney beans, undrained

STEPS IN PREPARATION:

1. Sauté onion and garlic in margarine in a large saucepan until tender.
2. Add salt and next 5 ingredients, stirring well.
3. Stir in tomato and beans. Simmer, uncovered, 10 to 15 minutes or until thoroughly heated.

Yield: 6 servings

Kidney beans are legumes, a class of vegetables that also includes pinto beans and other dried peas and beans. They're an especially good source of protein, are packed with fiber, and have no saturated fat or cholesterol. A ½-cup serving of red kidney beans provides as much iron as 6 ounces of lean red meat but only a trace of the fat.

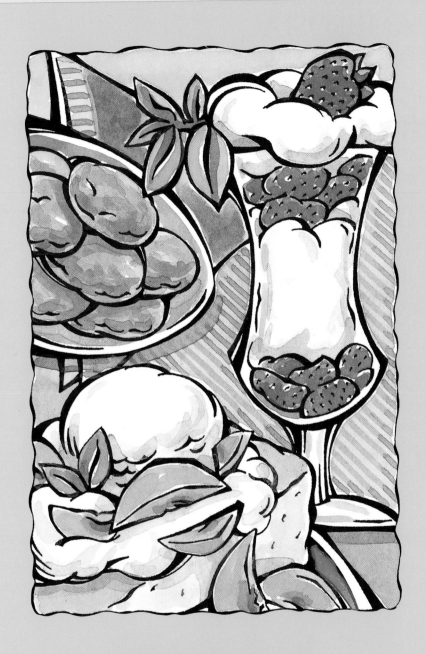

DESSERTS

AMBROSIA

Exchanges: 1 Fruit, ½ Fat

Serving Size: ½ cup	**Calories:** 86
Carbohydrate: 15 gm	**Fiber:** 2 gm
Protein: 1 gm	**Sodium:** 2 mg
Fat: 3 gm	**Cholesterol:** 0 mg

INGREDIENTS:

2 medium oranges, peeled
1 small banana, peeled
20 seedless green grapes,
   halved

¼ cup unsweetened shredded
   coconut

STEPS IN PREPARATION:

1. Section oranges, and cut into small pieces.
2. Cut banana into thin slices.
3. Combine orange slices, banana, grape halves, and coconut. Cover and chill.

Yield: 5 servings

Be sure to purchase unsweetened shredded coconut–¼ cup of unsweetened coconut contains about 5 grams of carbohydrate; ¼ cup of sweetened coconut contains 44 grams of carbohydrate.

SPICED FRUIT
Exchanges: 1 Fruit

Serving Size: ½ cup
Carbohydrate: 17 gm
Protein: 1 gm
Fat: trace

Calories: 91
Fiber: 4 gm
Sodium: 2 mg
Cholesterol: 0 mg

INGREDIENTS:

1 medium orange
1 (15¼-ounce) can pineapple chunks in juice
2 (16-ounce) cans pear halves in juice, drained

1 (16-ounce) can apricot halves in juice, drained
6 whole cloves
2 (2-inch) sticks cinnamon

STEPS IN PREPARATION:

1. Peel orange, reserving rind. Section orange; remove and discard seeds.
2. Drain pineapple, reserving juice.
3. Combine orange, pineapple, pear, and apricot in a large bowl; set aside.
4. Combine orange rind, reserved pineapple juice, cloves, and cinnamon in a small saucepan, stirring well. Bring to a boil; reduce heat, and simmer 5 minutes. Remove from heat.
5. Strain juice mixture, discarding rind and whole spices. Pour juice over fruit, tossing gently to combine. Cover and chill.

Yield: 12 servings

BAKED APPLES
Exchanges: 1 Fruit

Serving Size: 1 apple
Carbohydrate: 24 gm
Protein: 1 gm
Fat: trace

Calories: 98
Fiber: 2 gm
Sodium: 2 mg
Cholesterol: 0 mg

INGREDIENTS:

4 small cooking apples
1 cup water
Sugar substitute to equal 8
  teaspoons sugar*

1 tablespoon lemon juice
½ teaspoon ground cinnamon
½ teaspoon ground nutmeg

STEPS IN PREPARATION:

1. Wash and core apples; cut a small slice from the top and bottom of each apple. Place apples in a small baking dish.
2. Combine water and remaining ingredients; pour over apples. Bake at 350° for 45 minutes or until tender, basting every 15 minutes.

Yield: 4 servings

*See the sugar substitution chart on page 354.

Some of the best cooking apple varieties are Baldwin, Cortland, Granny Smith, Northern Spy, Rome Beauty, Winesap, and York Imperial.

SUGARLESS APPLE DESSERT

Exchanges: 2 Fruit

Serving Size: ½ cup
Carbohydrate: 35 gm
Protein: 4 gm
Fat: 1 gm

Calories: 166
Fiber: 1 gm
Sodium: 44 mg
Cholesterol: 0 mg

INGREDIENTS:

3 envelopes unflavored gelatin
1 (12-ounce) can unsweetened frozen apple juice concentrate, diluted with 1 can water

1 teaspoon ground cinnamon
½ teaspoon ground nutmeg
5 cups peeled, sliced apple
1 tablespoon reduced-calorie margarine

STEPS IN PREPARATION:

1. Combine first 4 ingredients in a large skillet, stirring well; let stand 1 minute. Cook over low heat 1 minute or until gelatin dissolves.
2. Add apple. Cover and cook over low heat 20 to 25 minutes or until tender, stirring frequently.
3. Add margarine; stir gently until margarine melts. Remove from heat. Cover and chill.
4. To serve, spoon mixture evenly into individual dessert dishes.

Yield: 5 servings

SPICED BAKED BANANAS

Exchanges: 1 Fruit

Serving Size: ½ banana
Carbohydrate: 11 gm
Protein: trace
Fat: trace

Calories: 43
Fiber: 1 gm
Sodium: 9 mg
Cholesterol: 0 mg

INGREDIENTS:

3 small, very ripe bananas, peeled
Vegetable cooking spray
4 teaspoons granulated brown sugar substitute

2 teaspoons grated lemon rind
½ teaspoon vanilla extract
⅛ teaspoon ground cinnamon

STEPS IN PREPARATION:

1. Cut bananas in half lenthwise; place bananas in an 11- x 7- x 2-inch baking dish coated with cooking spray.
2. Sprinkle with brown sugar substitute and remaining ingredients. Bake at 350° for 15 to 20 minutes or until thoroughly heated. Serve warm.

Yield: 6 servings

Keep ripe bananas an extra three to five days by refrigerating them. Or peel, mash, and freeze bananas, and store in airtight containers to use in baking. Even if bananas are past their prime, you can remove any brown portions and puree the rest to make banana bread, banana cake, or banana muffins.

BRANDIED ORANGES

Exchanges: 1 Fruit

Serving Size: ¼ cup
Carbohydrate: 18 gm
Protein: 1 gm
Fat: trace

Calories: 50
Fiber: 2 gm
Sodium: 2 mg
Cholesterol: 0 mg

INGREDIENTS:

3 large oranges, peeled and
  sectioned
⅓ cup raisins
¼ cup unsweetened orange
  juice

1 teaspoon brandy extract
¼ cup slivered almonds,
  toasted

STEPS IN PREPARATION:

1. Place orange sections in a medium bowl. Combine raisins, orange juice, and brandy extract; add to orange sections. Cover and chill overnight, stirring occasionally.
2. Sprinkle with almonds before serving.

Yield: 12 servings

CINNAMON ORANGES

Exchanges: 1 Fruit

Serving Size: ½ cup	**Calories:** 73
Carbohydrate: 18 gm	**Fiber:** 3 gm
Protein: 1 gm	**Sodium:** 2 mg
Fat: trace	**Cholesterol:** 0 mg

INGREDIENTS:

Sugar substitute to equal ¼ cup sugar*

¾ teaspoon ground cinnamon

¼ teaspoon ground cloves

4 medium oranges, peeled and thinly sliced

¼ cup water

½ teaspoon rum extract

STEPS IN PREPARATION:

1. Combine sugar substitute, cinnamon, and cloves in a small bowl.
2. Arrange half of orange slices in a 1-quart bowl; sprinkle with half of cinnamon mixture. Add remaining orange slices and remaining cinnamon mixture.
3. Combine water and rum extract; pour over orange mixture. Cover and chill overnight.
4. Spoon juice over oranges to moisten before serving.

Yield: 4 servings

*See the sugar substitution chart on page 354.

ORANGE DELIGHT

Exchanges: 1 Skim Milk

Serving Size: ¾ cup	**Calories:** 95
Carbohydrate: 14 gm	**Fiber:** 1 gm
Protein: 8 gm	**Sodium:** 267 mg
Fat: trace	**Cholesterol:** 3 mg

INGREDIENTS:

Whipped Topping (page 302)
2 cups 1% low-fat cottage cheese
2 (15¼-ounce) cans crushed pineapple in juice, well drained

1 (0.3-ounce) package sugar-free orange-flavored gelatin
Fresh mint sprigs (optional)

STEPS IN PREPARATION:

1. Spoon Whipped Topping into a medium bowl. Gently fold in cottage cheese, pineapple, and gelatin.
2. Spoon mixture evenly into individual dessert dishes, and garnish each serving with mint sprigs, if desired.

Yield: 8 servings

BAKED SPICED PEARS

Exchanges: 1 Fruit

Serving Size: ½ cup
Carbohydrate: 13 gm
Protein: trace
Fat: 1 gm

Calories: 56
Fiber: 3 gm
Sodium: 44 mg
Cholesterol: 0 mg

INGREDIENTS:

6 medium pears, peeled and
  sliced
¾ cup granulated brown
  sugar substitute
2 tablespoons crystallized
  ginger

1½ teaspoons rum extract
¼ teaspoon ground cinnamon
Dash of ground allspice
2 teaspoons reduced-calorie
  margarine

STEPS IN PREPARATION:

1. Arrange pear slices in an 11- x 7- x 2-inch baking dish.
2. Combine brown sugar substitute, ginger, rum extract, cinnamon, and allspice.
3. Sprinkle brown sugar mixture over pears; dot with margarine. Bake at 350° for 20 minutes. Serve warm or chilled.

Yield: 12 servings

Crystallized ginger is ginger that has been cooked in a sugar syrup and coated with coarse sugar. The amount of sugar in 2 tablespoons crystallized ginger has been calculated into this recipe and is acceptable for use in the diet plans of most people with diabetes.

PEACH CRUMB BAKE

Exchanges: 1 Fruit, ½ Fat

Serving Size: ½ cup	**Calories:** 75
Carbohydrate: 15 gm	**Fiber:** 2 gm
Protein: 1 gm	**Sodium:** 68 mg
Fat: 2 gm	**Cholesterol:** trace

INGREDIENTS:

2 cups sliced fresh peaches
Vegetable cooking spray
⅓ cup graham cracker
   crumbs

½ teaspoon ground cinnamon
⅛ teaspoon ground nutmeg
2 teaspoons reduced-calorie
   margarine, melted

STEPS IN PREPARATION:

1. Arrange peach slices in bottom of an 8-inch square baking dish coated with cooking spray.
2. Combine graham cracker crumbs, cinnamon, and nutmeg in a small bowl, stirring well. Add margarine, and stir until blended.
3. Sprinkle graham cracker crumb mixture over peaches, and bake at 350° for 30 minutes. Serve warm.

Yield: 4 servings

PINEAPPLE DESSERT

Exchanges: 1 Fruit

Serving Size: ½ cup
Carbohydrate: 15 gm
Protein: 3 gm
Fat: trace

Calories: 70
Fiber: 1 gm
Sodium: 35 mg
Cholesterol: 1 mg

INGREDIENTS:

1 (15¼-ounce) can crushed
   pineapple in juice
1 envelope unflavored gelatin
¼ teaspoon vanilla extract
½ cup instant nonfat dry
   milk powder

⅓ cup ice water
2 tablespoons lemon juice
Sugar substitute to equal 2
   teaspoons sugar*

STEPS IN PREPARATION:

1. Drain pineapple, reserving juice. Set pineapple aside. Add water,
   if necessary, to pineapple juice to yield 1 cup.
2. Combine juice mixture and gelatin in a small saucepan, stirring
   well; let stand 1 minute. Cook over low heat, stirring constantly,
   1 minute or until gelatin dissolves. Remove from heat, and stir in
   pineapple and vanilla. Cover and chill until mixture reaches the
   consistency of unbeaten egg white.
3. Combine milk powder and ice water in a medium bowl; beat at
   medium speed of an electric mixer until foamy. Add lemon juice;
   beat 3 to 4 minutes or until stiff peaks form, gradually adding
   sugar substitute.
4. Fold gelatin mixture into whipped milk mixture. Spoon evenly
   into 6 (6-ounce) custard cups or dessert dishes. Cover and chill.

Yield: 6 servings

*See the sugar substitution chart on page 354.

FRUIT MELBA

Exchanges: 1 Fruit

Serving Size: ¾ cup
Carbohydrate: 14 gm
Protein: 1 gm
Fat: trace

Calories: 59
Fiber: 2 gm
Sodium: 11 mg
Cholesterol: 0 mg

INGREDIENTS:

½ cup reduced-calorie
  cranberry juice
1 teaspoon cornstarch
4 drops almond extract

1 cup fresh or frozen
  unsweetened raspberries
3 cups cantaloupe balls

STEPS IN PREPARATION:

1. Combine cranberry juice and cornstarch in a small saucepan. Cook over medium heat, stirring constantly, until mixture is thick and bubbly.
2. Remove cranberry juice mixture from heat; stir in almond extract, and let cool.
3. Combine raspberries and cantaloupe balls; spoon ½ cup fruit mixture into each of 4 dessert dishes. Top evenly with cranberry juice mixture.

Yield: 4 servings

Featuring fruit as the main ingredient in desserts offers several nutritional benefits. Thanks to the natural sweetness of most fruit, you don't need to add much (if any) sugar. Fruit desserts also provide more vitamin, more fiber, and fewer calories than other types of desserts.

BAKED CUSTARD

Exchanges: ½ Skim Milk, ½ Fat

Serving Size: ½ cup
Carbohydrate: 8 gm
Protein: 6 gm
Fat: 2 gm

Calories: 76
Fiber: 0 gm
Sodium: 73 mg
Cholesterol: 77 mg

INGREDIENTS:

2 eggs
2 cups skim milk
Liquid sugar substitute to
  equal ⅓ cup sugar*

2 teaspoons vanilla extract

STEPS IN PREPARATION:

1. Lightly beat eggs in a small bowl; add milk, sugar substitute, and vanilla, and beat well.
2. Pour mixture evenly into 5 (6-ounce) custard cups, and place cups in a baking pan containing 1 inch hot water. Bake at 350° for 45 minutes or until a knife inserted in center comes out clean. Cover and chill thoroughly.

Yield: 5 servings

*See the sugar substitution chart on page 354.

Baked puddings thickened with eggs are often cooked in a baking pan filled with about 1 inch of water. The gentle heat from this cooking method helps to keep the pudding from breaking or curdling during cooking.

STRAWBERRY CRUNCH PARFAITS

Exchanges: 2 Starch, ½ Fruit, 1 Fat

Serving Size: 1 parfait
Carbohydrate: 41 gm
Protein: 7 gm
Fat: 7 gm

Calories: 245
Fiber: 3 gm
Sodium: 94 mg
Cholesterol: 0 mg

INGREDIENTS:

1¼ cups regular oats, uncooked
⅓ cup chopped pecans
2 tablespoons brown sugar
Vegetable cooking spray
3 tablespoons honey
2 tablespoons margarine, melted

2 teaspoons vanilla extract
1 teaspoon ground cinnamon
4 cups vanilla nonfat frozen yogurt
2 cups sliced fresh strawberries

STEPS IN PREPARATION:

1. Combine first 3 ingredients; place in a 13- x 9- x 2-inch baking pan coated with cooking spray. Combine honey and next 3 ingredients, stirring well; drizzle over oat mixture. Stir well. Bake at 350° for 20 minutes or until golden, stirring occasionally. Spoon oat mixture onto aluminum foil; let cool.
2. Spoon ¼ cup frozen yogurt into each of 8 (8-ounce) parfait glasses. Top each serving with 2 tablespoons strawberries and 2 tablespoons oat mixture; repeat layers with remaining yogurt, strawberries, and oat mixture.

Yield: 8 servings

STRAWBERRY MOUSSE

Exchanges: ½ Skim Milk

Serving Size: ½ cup
Carbohydrate: 7 gm
Protein: 4 gm
Fat: trace

Calories: 45
Fiber: trace
Sodium: 78 mg
Cholesterol: 1 mg

INGREDIENTS:

1 (0.3-ounce) package sugar-free strawberry-flavored gelatin
½ cup water
1½ cups sliced fresh strawberries

⅔ cup instant nonfat dry milk powder
6 ice cubes

STEPS IN PREPARATION:

1. Combine gelatin and water in a small saucepan, stirring well; let stand 1 minute. Cook over low heat, stirring constantly, 1 minute or until gelatin dissolves.
2. Combine gelatin mixture, strawberries, and milk powder in container of an electric blender; cover and process until smooth. Add ice cubes, one at a time, processing until blended.
3. Spoon mixture evenly into 6 parfait glasses. Cover and chill.

Yield: 6 servings

BERRY PUDDING
Exchanges: 1 Fruit

Serving Size: ½ cup
Carbohydrate: 17 gm
Protein: 1 gm
Fat: trace

Calories: 70
Fiber: 1 gm
Sodium: 46 mg
Cholesterol: 0 mg

INGREDIENTS:

3 cups fresh or frozen
  unsweetened berries,
  divided
1 cup water
3 tablespoons cornstarch
⅛ teaspoon salt

⅛ teaspoon ground
  cinnamon
Sugar substitute to equal 1
  cup sugar*
½ teaspoon vanilla or almond
  extract

STEPS IN PREPARATION:

1. Combine 1 cup berries, water, cornstarch, salt, and cinnamon in a
   medium saucepan. Cook over medium heat, stirring constantly,
   until mixture thickens.
2. Add remaining 2 cups berries, sugar substitute, and vanilla; stir
   well. Let cool before serving.

Yield: 6 servings

Note: Serve with Whipped Topping (page 302), if desired.

*See the sugar substitution chart on page 354.

BREAD PUDDING

Exchanges: 1½ Starch, 1 Fruit, ½ Skim Milk

Serving Size: ⅛ recipe
Carbohydrate: 42 gm
Protein: 9 gm
Fat: 2 gm

Calories: 215
Fiber: 2 gm
Sodium: 212 mg
Cholesterol: 58 mg

INGREDIENTS:

6 (1-ounce) slices whole
   wheat bread, toasted and
   cut into 1-inch pieces
Vegetable cooking spray
⅔ cup instant nonfat dry
   milk powder
½ cup sugar
Granulated sugar substitute
   to equal ½ cup sugar*

2 cups water
¼ teaspoon ground cinnamon
¼ teaspoon ground nutmeg
½ teaspoon vanilla extract
2 eggs
2 egg whites
½ cup raisins
1 cup chopped fresh peaches

STEPS IN PREPARATION:

1. Place bread in a 2-quart casserole coated with cooking spray.
2. Combine milk powder and next 8 ingredients. Add raisins and peaches; stir gently. Pour over bread.
3. Place casserole in a shallow pan; add hot water to pan to depth of 1 inch. Bake at 325° for 1 hour or until a knife inserted in center comes out clean.

Yield: 8 servings

*See the sugar substitution chart on page 354.

BAKED LEMON PUDDING

Exchanges: 1 Low-Fat Milk

Serving Size: ½ cup
Carbohydrate: 13 gm
Protein: 6 gm
Fat: 4 gm

Calories: 114
Fiber: 0 gm
Sodium: 199 mg
Cholesterol: 95 mg

INGREDIENTS:

3 eggs, separated
Sugar substitute to equal ½
  cup sugar*
¼ teaspoon salt
1½ cups skim milk
¼ cup plus 1 tablespoon
  all-purpose flour

¼ teaspoon grated lemon
  rind
⅓ cup plus 1 tablespoon
  lemon juice
2 tablespoons reduced-calorie
  margarine, melted

STEPS IN PREPARATION:

1. Combine egg whites, sugar substitute, and salt; beat at high speed of an electric mixer until soft peaks form.
2. Combine egg yolks, milk, and remaining ingredients; beat until smooth. Fold in egg white mixture.
3. Pour mixture evenly into 6 (6-ounce) custard cups. Place custard cups in a baking pan containing 1 inch hot water. Cover and bake at 325° for 1 hour or until a knife inserted in center comes out clean.

Yield: 6 servings

*See the sugar substitution chart on page 354.

ANGEL FOOD CAKE WITH CARAMEL SAUCE

Exchanges: 2½ Starch

Serving Size: 1 slice with sauce	**Calories:** 184
Carbohydrate: 41 gm	**Fiber:** 0 gm
Protein: 5 gm	**Sodium:** 105 mg
Fat: trace	**Cholesterol:** 1 mg

INGREDIENTS:

3 tablespoons brown sugar
1 tablespoon cornstarch
½ teaspoon instant espresso powder

1 cup skim milk
½ teaspoon vanilla extract
6 (2-ounce) slices angel food cake

STEPS IN PREPARATION:

1. Combine first 3 ingredients in a small saucepan, stirring well. Gradually stir in milk; bring to a boil, stirring constantly. Remove from heat; stir in vanilla.
2. Place cake slices on individual dessert plates. Top each serving with 2 tablespoons sauce. Serve immediately.

Yield: 6 servings

PUMPKIN-PECAN POUND CAKE

Exchanges: 2 Starch, 1 Fat

Serving Size: 1 slice	**Calories:** 213
Carbohydrate: 36 gm	**Fiber:** 1 gm
Protein: 3 gm	**Sodium:** 143 mg
Fat: 7 gm	**Cholesterol:** 0 mg

INGREDIENTS:

¾ cup margarine, softened
1½ cups firmly packed
  brown sugar
1 cup sugar
1¼ cups frozen egg substitute, thawed
1 (16-ounce) can pumpkin
⅓ cup unsweetened orange
  juice

3 cups all-purpose flour
2 teaspoons baking powder
½ teaspoon baking soda
¼ teaspoon salt
2 teaspoons pumpkin pie
  spice
¼ cup chopped pecans
Vegetable cooking spray

STEPS IN PREPARATION:

1. Beat margarine at medium speed of an electric mixer until creamy; gradually add sugars, beating well. Add egg substitute, and beat well.
2. Combine pumpkin and orange juice, stirring well. Combine flour and next 4 ingredients; add to margarine mixture alternately with pumpkin mixture, beginning and ending with flour mixture. Mix well after each addition.
3. Sprinkle pecans over bottom of a 10-inch tube pan coated with cooking spray. Spoon batter over pecans. Bake at 325° for 1 hour and 35 minutes or until a wooden pick inserted in center comes out clean. Cool in pan 10 minutes. Remove from pan. Cool completely on a wire rack.

Yield: 24 servings

HOMESTYLE APPLE PIE

Exchanges: ½ Starch, 1 Fruit, ½ Fat

Serving Size: ⅛ pie
Carbohydrate: 23 gm
Protein: 2 gm
Fat: 3 gm

Calories: 126
Fiber: 2 gm
Sodium: 338 mg
Cholesterol: 0 mg

INGREDIENTS:

Sugar substitute to equal ⅓ cup sugar*
1 tablespoon cornstarch
½ teaspoon grated lemon rind
1 teaspoon lemon juice
½ teaspoon ground cinnamon
¼ teaspoon ground nutmeg

4 small apples, peeled and sliced
1 cup all-purpose flour
1 teaspoon salt
¼ cup reduced-calorie margarine
3 tablespoons cold water

STEPS IN PREPARATION:

1. Combine first 7 ingredients. Place in a 9-inch deep-dish pieplate; set aside.
2. Combine flour and salt; cut in margarine with a pastry blender until mixture resembles coarse meal. Add water, stirring with a fork until dry ingredients are moistened.
3. Shape dough into a ball; roll out on a floured surface, and place on top of apple filling. Bake at 425° for 30 minutes or until lightly browned.

Yield: 8 servings

*See the sugar substitution chart on page 354.

APPLESAUCE-SPICE BUNDT CAKE

Exchanges: 2 Starch, 1 Fat

Serving Size: 1 slice	**Calories:** 181
Carbohydrate: 25 gm	**Fiber:** 1 gm
Protein: 2 gm	**Sodium:** 191 mg
Fat: 8 gm	**Cholesterol:** 20 mg

INGREDIENTS:

3 cups water, divided
1¼ cups raisins
2½ cups unsweetened
   applesauce
Sugar substitute to equal 1½
   cups sugar*
1 cup vegetable oil

3 eggs, lightly beaten
3 cups self-rising flour
¼ teaspoon baking soda
3 tablespoons ground
   cinnamon
2 tablespoons vanilla extract
Vegetable cooking spray

STEPS IN PREPARATION:

1. Combine 2½ cups water and raisins in a small Dutch oven; bring to a boil. Boil until water is absorbed. Remove from heat.
2. Add applesauce, sugar substitute, oil, eggs, and remaining ½ cup water. Stir until well blended.
3. Combine flour, soda, and cinnamon; gradually add to applesauce mixture, stirring after each addition. Stir in vanilla.
4. Spoon batter into a 10-inch Bundt pan coated with cooking spray. Bake at 350° for 40 to 45 minutes or until a wooden pick inserted in center comes out clean. Cool in pan 10 minutes; remove from pan, and cool completely on a wire rack.

Yield: 28 servings

*See the sugar substitution chart on page 354.

CHEESECAKE

Exchanges: ½ Starch, 1 Low-Fat Milk

Serving Size: 1 slice	**Calories:** 135
Carbohydrate: 19 gm	**Fiber:** 1 gm
Protein: 8 gm	**Sodium:** 290 mg
Fat: 4 gm	**Cholesterol:** 5 mg

INGREDIENTS:

2 teaspoons unflavored gelatin

2 tablespoons cold water

Sugar substitute to equal ⅓ cup sugar*

2½ cups 1% low-fat cottage cheese

1 teaspoon vanilla extract

1 (16-ounce) can cherries in water

2 teaspoons cornstarch

Sugar substitute to equal ¼ cup sugar*

⅛ teaspoon almond extract

6 drops red food coloring (optional)

14 (2½-inch) graham cracker squares, crushed

¼ cup reduced-calorie margarine, melted

Sugar substitute to equal 1 tablespoon sugar*

STEPS IN PREPARATION:

1. Sprinkle gelatin over cold water in a small saucepan; let stand 1 minute. Cook over low heat, stirring constantly, 2 minutes or until gelatin dissolves. Let cool.
2. Add sugar substitute to equal ⅓ cup sugar to cooled gelatin.
3. Combine cottage cheese and vanilla in container of an electric blender; cover and process until smooth. Gradually add gelatin mixture to cottage cheese mixture. Place cottage cheese mixture in a bowl, and chill 10 to 12 minutes or until slightly thickened, stirring occasionally.
4. Drain cherries, reserving liquid. Combine cornstarch and cherry liquid in a small saucepan; stir until smooth. Cook over medium heat, stirring constantly, until cornstarch mixture comes to a boil. Reduce heat, and cook 1 minute. Remove from heat, and stir in cherries.
5. Let cherry mixture cool slightly; add sugar substitute to equal ¼ cup sugar, almond extract, and red food coloring, if desired. Set cherry mixture aside.

6. Combine graham cracker crumbs, melted margarine, and sugar substitute to equal 1 tablespoon sugar. Press crumb mixture firmly into a 9-inch pieplate.
7. Spoon cottage cheese mixture into prepared crust; chill 15 minutes. Top with cherry mixture. Cover and chill at least 8 hours.

Yield: 12 servings

*See the sugar substitution chart on page 354.

Vary this basic cheesecake recipe by using fresh fruit instead of the canned cherry mixture. (The exchange values will remain the same.)

Try topping the cheesecake with 2 kiwifruit, peeled and thinly sliced, and 1 cup sliced fresh strawberries. Brush fruit lightly with ¼ cup melted low-sugar apple jelly.

Or arrange 1 cup thinly sliced fresh peaches and ½ cup fresh raspberries on the cake, and brush with melted low-sugar jelly.

INDIVIDUAL FRUIT CAKES

Exchanges: 1 Starch, ½ Fruit, 1 Fat

Serving Size: 1 cake	**Calories:** 147
Carbohydrate: 22 gm	**Fiber:** 2 gm
Protein: 2 gm	**Sodium:** 201 mg
Fat: 6 gm	**Cholesterol:** 0 mg

INGREDIENTS:

Liquid sugar substitute to equal 1½ cups sugar*
½ cup unsweetened orange juice
1 cup fresh cranberries, finely chopped or 1 cup sour cherries in water, drained and finely chopped
1 cup raisins
1 cup pecans, finely chopped
1 cup pineapple chunks in juice, drained and chopped
3 tablespoons reduced-calorie margarine, melted
1 tablespoon grated orange rind
1½ cups all-purpose flour
1 teaspoon baking soda
½ teaspoon salt
¼ teaspoon ground allspice
¼ teaspoon ground cinnamon
¼ teaspoon ground nutmeg
Vegetable cooking spray

STEPS IN PREPARATION:

1. Pour sugar substitute and orange juice over chopped cranberries; let stand 1 hour.
2. Add raisins, pecans, pineapple, margarine, and orange rind to cranberry mixture.
3. Combine flour and next 5 ingredients; add dry ingredients to fruit mixture, and stir until well blended.
4. Spoon mixture into 16 muffin cups coated with cooking spray. Bake at 325° for 30 to 35 minutes or until lightly browned.

Yield: 16 individual cakes

*See the sugar substitution chart on page 354.

RAISIN CAKE

Exchanges: 2 Starch, 1 Fat

Serving Size: 1 slice
Carbohydrate: 37 gm
Protein: 4 gm
Fat: 4 gm

Calories: 197
Fiber: 1 gm
Sodium: 177 mg
Cholesterol: 15 mg

INGREDIENTS:

2 cups water
1 cup reduced-calorie margarine
1 (15-ounce) package raisins
Sugar substitute to equal 1 cup sugar*
2 teaspoons baking soda
¼ cup warm water

2 eggs, lightly beaten
4½ cups all-purpose flour
½ teaspoon baking powder
1 teaspoon ground cloves
1 teaspoon ground allspice
1 teaspoon ground cinnamon
Vegetable cooking spray

STEPS IN PREPARATION:

1. Bring 2 cups water to a boil in a large saucepan; stir in margarine and raisins. Let stand, uncovered, 5 minutes. Let raisin mixture cool. Stir in sugar substitute.
2. Dissolve soda in ¼ cup warm water; add to raisin mixture, stirring well. Stir in eggs.
3. Combine flour and next 4 ingredients; gradually add to raisin mixture, stirring after each addition.
4. Spoon batter into a 10-inch Bundt pan coated with cooking spray. Bake at 350° for 50 minutes to 1 hour or until a wooden pick inserted in center comes out clean. Cool cake in pan 10 minutes. Remove from pan; let cool on a wire rack.

Yield: 24 servings

*See the sugar substitution chart on page 354.

ORANGE STREUSEL CAKE

Exchanges: 1½ Starch, ½ Fat

Serving Size: 1 slice	**Calories:** 147
Carbohydrate: 25 gm	**Fiber:** 1 gm
Protein: 4 gm	**Sodium:** 167 mg
Fat: 3 gm	**Cholesterol:** 15 mg

INGREDIENTS:

1 package dry yeast
Sugar substitute to equal ⅓ cup sugar, divided*
½ cup warm water (105° to 115°)
1 egg
2¾ cups all-purpose flour, divided
2 tablespoons reduced-calorie margarine, melted

2 tablespoons low-sugar orange marmalade
½ teaspoon salt
Vegetable cooking spray
¼ cup reduced-calorie margarine, melted
1 tablespoon grated orange rind
1 tablespoon unsweetened orange juice

STEPS IN PREPARATION:

1. Dissolve yeast and one-fifth of sugar substitute in water; let stand 5 minutes. Add egg, beating well.
2. Add 1 cup flour and next 3 ingredients. Beat until smooth. Add 1¼ cups flour to make a soft dough.
3. Turn dough out onto a lightly floured surface; knead until smooth and elastic. Place in a bowl coated with cooking spray, turning to grease top.
4. Cover and let rise in a warm place (85°), free from drafts, 50 minutes or until doubled in bulk. Punch down. Press into a 9-inch round pan coated with cooking spray.
5. Combine remaining sugar substitute, remaining ½ cup flour, ¼ cup margarine, orange rind, and juice; stir well, and sprinkle over dough. Cover and let rise in a warm place, free from drafts, 25 minutes or until doubled in bulk. Bake at 375° for 25 minutes.

Yield: 12 servings

*See the sugar substitution chart on page 354.

TASTY PINEAPPLE CAKE

Exchanges: 1½ Starch, 1 Fat

Serving Size: 1 slice
Carbohydrate: 26 gm
Protein: 3 gm
Fat: 5 gm

Calories: 158
Fiber: 1 gm
Sodium: 219 mg
Cholesterol: 31 mg

INGREDIENTS:

½ cup reduced-calorie
  margarine
Sugar substitute to equal 2¼
  cups sugar*
2 eggs
1½ cups all-purpose flour
1 teaspoon baking powder

½ teaspoon baking soda
¼ teaspoon salt
½ cup skim milk
4 slices canned pineapple in
  juice, drained
1 tablespoon all-purpose flour
Vegetable cooking spray

STEPS IN PREPARATION:

1. Beat margarine at medium speed of an electric mixer until creamy; gradually add sugar substitute, beating well. Add eggs, one at a time, beating well.
2. Combine 1½ cups flour, baking powder, soda, and salt. Add to creamed mixture alternately with milk, beginning and ending with flour mixture. Beat at low speed after each addition. Cut pineapple into ½-inch pieces; toss with 1 tablespoon flour, and gently fold into batter.
3. Spoon batter into a 6-cup Bundt pan coated with cooking spray. Bake at 350° for 35 to 40 minutes or until a wooden pick inserted in center comes out clean.
4. Remove cake from oven; let stand 5 minutes. Remove cake from pan, and cool completely on a wire rack.

Yield: 12 servings

*See the sugar substitution chart on page 354.

ALMOND COOKIES

Exchanges: ½ Starch

Serving Size: 1 cookie
Carbohydrate: 7 gm
Protein: 1 gm
Fat: 2 gm

Calories: 51
Fiber: trace
Sodium: 68 mg
Cholesterol: 13 mg

INGREDIENTS:

¼ cup plus 2 tablespoons
  reduced-calorie margarine
Sugar substitute to equal ¼
  cup sugar*
1 egg yolk
½ teaspoon almond extract

¼ teaspoon vanilla extract
¼ teaspoon lemon extract
1 cup all-purpose flour
½ teaspoon baking powder
⅛ teaspoon salt

STEPS IN PREPARATION:

1. Beat margarine at medium speed of an electric mixer until creamy; gradually add sugar substitute, beating well. Add egg yolk and extracts; beat well.
2. Combine flour, baking powder, and salt; add to creamed mixture, beating well.
3. Shape dough into 1-inch balls; place 2 inches apart on nonstick cookie sheets. Press each with a fork to flatten.
4. Bake at 300° for 20 minutes or until edges begin to brown. Remove cookies to wire racks, and let cool completely.

Yield: 15 cookies

*See the sugar substitution chart on page 354.

APPLESAUCE COOKIES

Exchanges: 1 Starch, ½ Fat

Serving Size: 2 cookies
Carbohydrate: 15 gm
Protein: 2 gm
Fat: 3 gm

Calories: 87
Fiber: 2 gm
Sodium: 208 mg
Cholesterol: 10 mg

INGREDIENTS:

1¾ cups sifted cake flour
1 teaspoon baking soda
½ teaspoon salt
1 teaspoon ground cinnamon
½ teaspoon ground nutmeg
½ teaspoon ground cloves
½ cup reduced-calorie
  margarine

Liquid sugar substitute to
  equal ½ cup sugar*
1 teaspoon vanilla extract
1 egg
1 cup unsweetened
  applesauce
1 cup wheat bran cereal
⅓ cup raisins

STEPS IN PREPARATION:

1. Sift together first 6 ingredients.
2. Combine margarine, sugar substitute, vanilla, and egg; beat well.
3. Add flour mixture and applesauce alternately to creamed mixture, beating well after each addition. Fold in bran cereal and raisins.
4. Drop cookie dough by level tablespoonfuls, 1 inch apart, onto nonstick cookie sheets.
5. Bake at 375° for 10 to 12 minutes or until lightly browned. Remove to wire racks, and let cool completely.

Yield: 3 dozen cookies

*See the sugar substitution chart on page 354.

CINNAMON COOKIES

Exchanges: ½ Starch

Serving Size: 3 cookies
Carbohydrate: 10 gm
Protein: 1 gm
Fat: 3 gm

Calories: 73
Fiber: 1 gm
Sodium: 98 mg
Cholesterol: 0 mg

INGREDIENTS:

1 cup all-purpose flour
¼ teaspoon baking powder
¼ cup plus 1 tablespoon reduced-calorie margarine
2 teaspoons vanilla extract

Liquid sugar substitute to equal ⅓ cup sugar*
1 tablespoon unsweetened orange juice
1 teaspoon ground cinnamon

STEPS IN PREPARATION:

1. Combine flour and baking powder in a medium bowl.
2. Combine margarine and vanilla; beat well. Add flour mixture to creamed mixture.
3. Combine sugar substitute and orange juice. Add juice mixture to flour mixture, stirring well.
4. Sprinkle cinnamon over dough, and knead to make a streaked appearance. Shape dough into 30 (½-inch) balls; place on nonstick cookie sheets. Flatten balls with a fork dipped in cold water.
5. Bake at 350° for 12 to 15 minutes or until lightly browned. Remove to wire racks, and let cool completely.

Yield: 2½ dozen cookies

*See the sugar substitution chart on page 354.

LEMON-COCONUT COOKIES

Exchanges: 1 Starch, 1 Fat

Serving Size: 3 cookies
Carbohydrate: 12 gm
Protein: 2 gm
Fat: 4 gm

Calories: 94
Fiber: 1 gm
Sodium: 162 mg
Cholesterol: 10 mg

INGREDIENTS:

½ cup reduced-calorie margarine
Liquid sugar substitute to equal ½ cup sugar*
1 tablespoon water
1 tablespoon grated lemon rind
1 tablespoon lemon juice

1 teaspoon vanilla extract
1 egg
½ cup unsweetened shredded coconut
2 cups all-purpose flour
1 teaspoon baking powder
½ teaspoon salt

STEPS IN PREPARATION:

1. Beat margarine at medium speed of an electric mixer until creamy; gradually add sugar substitute, beating well.
2. Add water and next 4 ingredients; beat until well blended. Add coconut, stirring well.
3. Combine flour, baking powder, and salt. Add to creamed mixture, beating well at low speed.
4. Shape dough into a 2-inch diameter roll; wrap in wax paper. Chill until firm. Cut into 54 thin slices, and place on nonstick cookie sheets.
5. Bake at 375° for 10 to 12 minutes or until lightly browned. Remove to wire racks, and let cool completely.

Yield: 4½ dozen cookies

*See the sugar substitution chart on page 354.

OATMEAL COOKIES

Exchanges: ½ Starch, ½ Fat

Serving Size: 2 cookies	**Calories:** 80
Carbohydrate: 11 gm	**Fiber:** 1 gm
Protein: 2 gm	**Sodium:** 114 mg
Fat: 3 gm	**Cholesterol:** 0 mg

INGREDIENTS:

1½ cups all-purpose flour
½ teaspoon baking soda
¼ teaspoon salt
1½ cups quick-cooking oats, uncooked

Sugar substitute to equal ½ cup sugar*
¾ cup reduced-calorie margarine, softened
3 tablespoons cold water

STEPS IN PREPARATION:

1. Combine first 5 ingredients in a large bowl. Cut margarine into dry mixture with a pastry blender until mixture resembles coarse meal. Sprinkle cold water evenly over surface; stir with a fork until dry ingredients are moistened.
2. Roll dough to ¼-inch thickness on wax paper. Cut into 46 rounds with a 1-inch cookie cutter. Place cookies on nonstick cookie sheets.
3. Bake at 375° for 12 minutes or until lightly browned. Remove to wire racks, and let cool completely.

Yield: 46 cookies

*See the sugar substitution chart on page 354.

VANILLA COOKIES

Exchanges: ½ Starch

Serving Size: 1 cookie
Carbohydrate: 5 gm
Protein: 1 gm
Fat: 1 gm

Calories: 32
Fiber: trace
Sodium: 30 mg
Cholesterol: 0 mg

INGREDIENTS:

⅓ cup margarine, softened
⅔ cup sugar
¼ cup frozen egg substitute, thawed
2 teaspoons vanilla extract
2 cups plus 1 tablespoon all-purpose flour

½ teaspoon baking soda
¼ teaspoon salt
¾ cup crisp rice cereal
Vegetable cooking spray

STEPS IN PREPARATION:

1. Beat margarine at medium speed of an electric mixer until creamy; gradually add sugar, beating well. Add egg substitute and vanilla; beat well.
2. Combine flour, soda, and salt. Gradually add flour mixture to creamed mixture; mix well. Stir in cereal.
3. Divide dough into 2 equal portions; roll each into an 8- x 1½-inch log. Wrap logs in wax paper. Freeze until firm.
4. Unwrap logs, and cut into ¼-inch slices. Place 1 inch apart on cookie sheets coated with cooking spray. Bake at 350° for 6 to 8 minutes or until lightly browned. Remove to wire racks, and let cool completely.

Yield: 64 cookies

DATE-OAT BARS

Exchanges: 1 Starch, 1 Fat

Serving Size: 1 bar
Carbohydrate: 14 gm
Protein: 2 gm
Fat: 4 gm

Calories: 95
Fiber: 2 gm
Sodium: 48 mg
Cholesterol: 0 mg

INGREDIENTS:

1 (8-ounce) package pitted dates, chopped
1 tablespoon all-purpose flour
½ cup water
¾ cup unsweetened shredded coconut
½ cup reduced-calorie margarine
Sugar substitute to equal ½ cup sugar*
2½ cups quick-cooking oats, uncooked
½ teaspoon vanilla extract
Vegetable cooking spray

STEPS IN PREPARATION:

1. Combine chopped dates and flour in a large bowl. Toss lightly to coat.
2. Place water in a 1-cup glass measure; microwave at HIGH for 2 to 3 minutes or until boiling. Pour water over dates.
3. Add coconut, margarine, and sugar substitute to date mixture, stirring well. Microwave at HIGH for 2 to 3 minutes or until thickened, stirring at 1-minute intervals. Add oats and vanilla to date mixture, stirring well.
4. Spoon mixture into a 9-inch square pan coated with cooking spray; press evenly into bottom of pan. Cover and chill.
5. Cut into 24 bars, and store in an airtight container in refrigerator.

Yield: 2 dozen bars

*See the sugar substitution chart on page 354.

STRAWBERRY THUMBPRINT COOKIES

Exchanges: ½ Starch

Serving Size: 1 cookie
Carbohydrate: 8 gm
Protein: 1 gm
Fat: 2 gm

Calories: 52
Fiber: trace
Sodium: 34 mg
Cholesterol: 0 mg

INGREDIENTS:

1 (17.5-ounce) package
  regular chocolate chip
  cookie mix
1 cup regular oats, uncooked
⅓ cup water
1 teaspoon vanilla extract

1 egg white
Vegetable cooking spray
¼ cup plus 2 teaspoons
  no-sugar-added strawberry
  spread

STEPS IN PREPARATION:

1. Combine first 5 ingredients; drop by 2 level teaspoonfuls 1 inch apart onto cookie sheets coated with cooking spray.
2. Press center of each cookie with thumb, making an indentation; fill with ¼ teaspoon strawberry spread. Bake at 375° for 10 minutes or until lightly browned. Remove to wire racks, and let cool completely.

Yield: 4½ dozen cookies

PINEAPPLE-ORANGE FROZEN YOGURT

Exchanges: ½ Fruit, ½ Starch

Serving Size: ½ cup	**Calories:** 64
Carbohydrate: 13 gm	**Fiber:** trace
Protein: 3 gm	**Sodium:** 26 mg
Fat: trace	**Cholesterol:** 1 mg

INGREDIENTS:

1 envelope unflavored gelatin
¼ cup cold water
2 (8-ounce) cartons plain nonfat yogurt
1 (8-ounce) can pineapple chunks in juice, drained

1 (6-ounce) can frozen orange juice concentrate, thawed and undiluted
⅓ cup sugar
¾ cup cold water

STEPS IN PREPARATION:

1. Sprinkle gelatin over ¼ cup cold water in a small saucepan; let stand 1 minute. Cook over low heat, stirring until gelatin dissolves, about 2 minutes.
2. Place gelatin mixture, yogurt, and remaining ingredients in container of an electric blender; cover and process until smooth.
3. Pour mixture into freezer container of a 4-quart hand-turned or electric freezer. Freeze according to manufacturer's instructions.

Yield: 14 servings

CHOCOLATE-CHERRY SQUARES

Exchanges: 1 Starch, 1 Fruit

Serving Size: 1 square
Carbohydrate: 31 gm
Protein: 6 gm
Fat: 0 gm

Calories: 145
Fiber: 2 gm
Sodium: 100 mg
Cholesterol: 0 mg

INGREDIENTS:

1 cup diced, pitted fresh
  sweet cherries
2 tablespoons rum
6 cups sugar-free, fat-free
  chocolate ice cream,
  softened

Vegetable cooking spray
2 teaspoons grated semisweet
  chocolate

STEPS IN PREPARATION:

1. Fold cherries and rum into ice cream. Spread mixture evenly
into an 8-inch square pan coated with cooking spray. Cover and
freeze until firm.
2. Sprinkle with grated chocolate, and cut into squares. Serve
immediately.

Yield: 9 servings

SUGAR SUBSTITUTIONS

Brand Name of Sugar Substitute	Amount of Sugar Substitute	Equivalent Amount of Sugar
Adolph's	2 shakes of jar	1 teaspoon sugar
	¼ teaspoon	1 tablespoon sugar
	1 teaspoon	¼ cup sugar
	2½ teaspoons	⅔ cup sugar
	1 tablespoon	¾ cup sugar
	4 teaspoons	1 cup sugar
Equal*	1 packet	2 teaspoons sugar
NutraSweet Spoonful	1 teaspoon	1 teaspoon sugar
Sugar Twin	1 teaspoon	1 teaspoon sugar
Sugar Twin, Brown	1 teaspoon	1 teaspoon brown sugar
Sweet Magic	1 packet	2 teaspoons sugar
Sweet'ner	1 packet	2 teaspoons sugar
Sweet 'N Low	¹⁄₁₀ teaspoon	1 teaspoon sugar
	1 packet	2 teaspoons sugar
	⅓ teaspoon	1 tablespoon sugar
	1½ teaspoons	¼ cup sugar
	1 tablespoon	½ cup sugar
	2 tablespoons	1 cup sugar
Sweet 'N Low, Brown	¼ teaspoon	1 tablespoon brown sugar
	1 teaspoon	¼ cup brown sugar
	4 teaspoons	1 cup brown sugar
Sweet One	1 packet	2 teaspoons sugar
	3 packets	¼ cup sugar
	4 packets	⅓ cup sugar
	6 packets	½ cup sugar
	12 packets	1 cup sugar

Brand Name of Sugar Substitute	Amount of Sugar Substitute	Equivalent Amount of Sugar
Fasweet (liquid)	⅛ teaspoon	1 teaspoon sugar
	¼ teaspoon	2 teaspoons sugar
	⅓ teaspoon	1 tablespoon sugar
	1 tablespoon	½ cup sugar
	2 tablespoons	1 cup sugar
Sucaryl (liquid)	⅛ teaspoon	1 teaspoon sugar
	⅓ teaspoon	1 tablespoon sugar
	½ teaspoon	4 teaspoons sugar
	1½ teaspoons	¼ cup sugar
	1 tablespoon	½ cup sugar
Superose (liquid)	4 drops	1 teaspoon sugar
	⅛ teaspoon	2 teaspoons sugar
	¼ teaspoon	1 tablespoon sugar
	1½ teaspoons	½ cup sugar
	1 tablespoon	1 cup sugar
Sweet-10 (liquid)	10 drops	1 teaspoon sugar
	½ teaspoon	4 teaspoons sugar
	1½ teaspoons	¼ cup sugar
	1 tablespoon	½ cup sugar
	2 tablespoons	1 cup sugar
Zero-Cal (liquid)	10 drops	1 teaspoon sugar
	30 drops	1 tablespoon sugar
	¾ teaspoon	2 tablespoons sugar
	1 tablespoon	½ cup sugar
	2 tablespoons	1 cup sugar

Note: Sugar equivalents for various brand names of sugar substitutes are listed for your convenience and are not an endorsement of any product.

*Use only after cooking or in uncooked dishes.

RECIPE INDEX

Pork. *See also* Ham.
Chop Dinner, Pork, 150
Chops, Creole Pork, 151
Chops with Apples, Pork, 149
Sweet-and-Sour Pork, 152
Potatoes
Baked Potatoes, Twice-, 214
Casserole, Potato, 213
Casserole, Potato-Cheese, 216
Frittata, Cheddar-Potato, 88
Hash Brown Potatoes, 211
New Potatoes, Herbed, 212
Omelet, Potato-Mushroom, 93
Pancakes, Potato, 74
Salad, Potato, 272
Salad, Tarragon Potato, 273
Scalloped Potatoes, 215
Soup, Creamed Potato, 307
Sweet Potato Casserole, 217
Sweet Potatoes, Spiced, 218
Puddings. *See also* Custards.
Berry Pudding, 331
Bread Pudding, 332
Corn Pudding, 210
Lemon Pudding, Baked, 333
Pumpkin-Pecan Pound Cake, 335

Q
Quiche, Zucchini, 100

R
Raisins
Cake, Raisin, 341
Muffins, Raisin-Bran, 58
Oatmeal with Raisins and
Cinnamon, 78
Salad, Carrot-Raisin, 264
Rice
Baked Cheese and Rice, 187
Baked Rice, 186

Black Beans and Rice, 197
Black-Eyed Peas with Rice, 188
Casserole, Broccoli and Rice, 226
Casserole, Chicken and Rice, 159
Casserole, Egg-Rice, 91
Casserole, Vegetable-Rice, 195
Casserole, Wild Rice, 194
Chicken with Rice, Baked, 168
"Fried" Rice, Ham, 189
Holiday Rice, 190
Mexican Rice, 191
Parslied Rice, 193
Pilaf, Tuna, 119
Red Beans and Rice, 196
Spice Rice, Hint-of-, 192
Rolls. *See also* Breads.
Cinnamon Rolls, 70
Parker House Rolls, 69

S
Salad Dressings
Cucumber Dressing, 278
French Dressing, 279
Herb Dressing, 280
Italian Dressing, 281
Mandarin Dressing, 282
Thousand Island Dressing, 283
Vinegar Salad Dressing, 284
Yogurt-Fruit Salad Dressing, 285
Zero Salad Dressing, 286
Salads
Aspic, Tomato, 274
Bean Salad, Green, 263
Beet Salad, Pickled, 262
Caesar Salad, 261
Carrot-Raisin Salad, 264
Cauliflower Salad, Chilled, 265
Chef's Salad, 276
Chicken Salad, 156
Coleslaw, 267

Squash. *See also* Zucchini.
  Baked Squash with Rosemary, 240
  Butternut Squash, Stuffed, 244
  Casserole, Squash, 241
  Dilly Squash, 239
  Mix with Chicken, Squash, 175
Stew, Beef, 145
Strawberries
  Cookies, Strawberry Thumbprint, 351
  Mousse, Strawberry, 330
  Parfaits, Strawberry Crunch, 329
  Salad, Strawberry, 260
  Sauce, Strawberry, 301
  Shake, Strawberry-Orange, 52

T
Tea, Lemon-Orange, 41
Tea Mix, Low-Calorie Spiced, 40
Tea, Spiced Hot, 39
Tomatoes
  Aspic, Tomato, 274
  Baked Tomatoes, 247
  Bouillon, Tomato, 308
  Cacciatore, Chicken, 165
  Salsa, 296
  Sauce, Meatless Tomato, 297
  Sauce, Vermicelli with Tomato, 204
  Scalloped Tomatoes, 248
  Stewed Tomatoes, 245
  Stuffed Tomatoes, Spinach-, 246
  Stuffed Tomatoes, Turkey-, 184
Toppings. *See* Sauces and Toppings.
Tortilla Casserole, Chicken, 160
Tostada with Salsa, Chicken, 176
Tuna
  Creole, Tuna, 115
  Pilaf, Tuna, 119
  Salad, Tuna, 116
  Stir-Fried Tuna, 118
  Toss, Spicy Tuna Pasta, 117

Turkey
  Hash, Turkey, 183
  Salad, Chef's, 276
  Salad, Turkey, 277
  Tomatoes, Turkey-Stuffed, 184
Turnip Greens, 249

V
Veal Parmigiana, 147
Veal Scallopini, 148
Vegetables. *See also* specific types.
  Casserole, Chicken and
    Vegetable, 161
  Casserole, Mixed Vegetable, 250
  Casserole, Vegetable-Rice, 195
  Dinner, Six-Layer Beef, 137
  Kabobs, Beef and Vegetable, 138
  Marinated Garden Vegetables, 252
  Pasta in Cheese Sauce, Vegetables
    and, 203
  Pizzas, Vegetarian, 99
  Pot Roast with Vegetables, 146
  Salad, Marinated Vegetable, 270
  Snapper, Vegetable-Topped, 114
  Soup, Vegetable-Cheese, 309
  Stir-Fried Vegetables, 251

Y
Yogurt
  Frozen Yogurt, Pineapple-Orange, 352
  Salad Dressing, Yogurt-Fruit, 285
  Shake, Orange-Yogurt, 51

Z
Zucchini
  Baked Zucchini Squash, 242
  Bread, Zucchini-Orange, 64
  Quiche, Zucchini, 100
  Sautéed Zucchini, 243
  Soup, Zucchini, 310

SUBJECT INDEX

A
Alcohol, in cooking, 141
American Diabetes Association,
    the, 4, 12
American Dietetic Association,
    The, 4, 12
American Heart Association
    guidelines for beef, 137
    guidelines for cholesterol, 120
    guidelines for eggs, 85
Apples, varieties of, 318

B
Bananas, storage of, 320
Beans
    green, 207, 229, 263
    kidney, 314
Beef
    American Heart Association
        guidelines for, 137
    ground, fat content of, 131
    lean cuts of, 140
Body Mass Index (BMI) *See also*
    Weight, 8, 9
Breadcrumbs, 80
Broccoli, nutrient content of, 225

C
Cabbage, selection and storage
    of, 267
Calories
    daily intake, 10
    in exchange values, 13
    in free foods, 30
Carbohydrate, 10, 11, 316
    counting, 11, 12
    exchange values, 13, 20–21

Carrots, vitamin A content of, 230
Chicken, fat content of, 167
Cholesterol
    daily intake, 10, 120, 137
    reducing intake, 10, 120, 307
Coconut, carbohydrate
    in, 316
Combination foods, values
    for, 32, 33
Corn, 207, 209
Cornstarch, in sauces, 293
Cranberry juice cocktail, 46

D
Diabetes mellitus
    meal plan for, 11, 12
    types of, 6

E
Eggplant
    preparation of, 232
    varieties of, 96
Eggs
    American Heart Association
        guidelines for, 85
    storage of, 87, 91, 94
Egg substitutes, 88
Exchange lists
    explanation of, 12, 13
    Fat, 28–29
    Free foods, 30–31
    Fruit, 17–18
    Meat and meat substitutes, 24–27
    Milk, 19
    Other carbohydrates, 20–21
    Starch, 14–16
    Vegetable, 22–23

365

F

Fast foods, values for, 34
Fat
  daily intake, 6, 7, 10, 11
  defatting stock, 292
  exchange list, 28–29
  exchange values, 12, 13
  low-fat snack products, 296
  monounsaturated, 11, 28
  polyunsaturated, 28–29
  reducing intake, 307
  saturated, 11, 28–29, 120, 137
Fiber
  guidelines for, 58
  increasing intake of, 75
  insoluble, 58
Fish
  oils, omega-3 fatty
    acids, 106
  preparation of, 110
  storage of, 102
  tuna, varieties of, 116
Flour, in sauces, 293
Food Group Pyramid,
    Jenny Craig, 10
Free foods, 30–31
Fruit
  exchange list, 17–18
  in desserts, 327, 339
  in salads, 254

G

Garnishes, 39, 312
Ginger, crystallized, 324
Gravy, 292

H

Ham, reduced-fat, 154
Herbs, 171, 312
High blood pressure, 6, 7, 9

J

Journal, daily, 9
Juice
  as cooking liquid, 186
  cranberry juice cocktail, 46
  substitutions, 43
  tomato juice, 308

L

Labels, 35
Legumes, nutrient content of, 188, 314
Lifestyle, 4, 6, 7, 9
  daily journal, 9

M

Measuring foods, 12, 35
Meat and meat substitutes,
    exchange list, 24–27
Milk
  exchange list, 19
  use in low-fat recipes, 307

N

Nutritional analysis, 36
Nutrition Basics, 10–11

O

Oats, use in recipes, 78
Okra, selection and storage of, 236
Onions, storage of, 211

P

Pasta
  storage of, 201
  vermicelli, 204
Peas, 207
Potatoes
  nutrient content of, 213
  storage of, 211, 218
  sweet, 218

Poultry. *See* Chicken or Turkey.
Protein, exchange values, 13
Pudding, baking, 328

R
Registered dietitian, 4, 8, 11, 32
Rice, cooking, 186, 191

S
Salads, in meal planning, 254, 266
Salt. *See* Sodium.
Sauces, thickening, 293
Seasoning, 292
Snacks
    low-fat products, 296
    tortilla chips, 294, 296
Sodium
    in vegetables, 209, 229, 263, 308
    reducing, 174, 209, 229, 263, 308
Soy sauce, 174
Spices, 31, 71
Squash, selection of, 239
Starch, exchange list, 14–16
Sugar
    guidelines, 11
    substitutes for, 354–355
Sugar substitutes, 354–355
Sweeteners. *See* Sugar Substitutes.

T
Tomato juice, 308
Tortilla chips, 294
Turkey
    smaller cuts of, 277
    storage of, 183

U
U.S. Department of Agriculture
    (USDA), 71
    Food Guide Pyramid, 10

V
Veal, fat content of, 147
Vegetables. *See also* specific types.
    exchange list, 22–23
    storage of, 207, 211, 236, 267
Vitamin A
    in broccoli, 225
    in carrots, 230
Vitamin C
    in broccoli, 225
    in juice, 46

W
Weight. *See also* Body Mass Index.
    control, 6, 7, 9, 11
Wheat bran cereal, 58
Worcestershire sauce, 174

Y
Yogurt, fat content of, 51

ACKNOWLEDGMENTS

Betty E. Darnell, M.S., R.D., Director of Nutrition, General Clinical Research Center, School of Medicine, University Hospital, University of Alabama at Birmingham

Registered Dietitians and staff of the Department of Food and Nutrition Services, University Hospital, University of Alabama at Birmingham:

- Charlotte Knight Beeker
- Mandy Berry
- Sandra Dillon, M.S., R.D.
- Lynn Epps Eden, M.S., R.D.
- Yolanda Guyton
- Linda Harbour, R.D.
- Susan Hommerson, M.S., R.D.
- Sarah Hood, M.S., R.D.
- Elizabeth Ivins
- Margaret Stewart McDonald, R.D.
- Cassandra C. Mills
- Laura Moore
- Lisa Mullins, M.S., R.D.
- Kimberly Garrison Nunn
- Margaret Palmer, M.S., R.D.
- Bessie Rawls
- Debra Simerly, M.S., R.D.
- Cynthia Wren

We would also like to acknowledge those at Jenny Craig International who believe that healthful nutrition can reduce the incidence of disease and improve many health conditions, including diabetes:

- C. Joseph LaBonté, President, CEO
- Michael Jeub, Sr.V.P., CFO
- Les Koll, Sr.V.P., Marketing
- Jan Strode, V.P., Corp. Communications
- Lisa Talamini Jones, RD, Dir., Program Development
- Daren Hillebrandt, Dir., Product Development

FAVORITE RECIPES

Recipe Title   *page*

_____   _____

_____   _____

_____   _____

_____   _____

_____   _____

_____   _____

_____   _____

_____   _____

_____   _____

_____   _____

_____   _____

_____   _____

_____   _____

_____   _____

_____   _____

_____   _____

_____   _____

_____   _____

_____   _____

_____   _____

Recipe Title *page*

NOTES

NOTES